Losing It?

Losing It?

The Psychology of Losing Weight and Never Finding it Again

John Whitney

iUniverse, Inc.
New York Lincoln Shanghai

Losing It?
The Psychology of Losing Weight and Never Finding it Again

iUniverse, Inc.

For information address:
iUniverse, Inc.
2021 Pine Lake Road, Suite 100
Lincoln, NE 68512
www.iuniverse.com

ISBN: 0-595-31573-9

Printed in the United States of America

To Burt and Deb for all of your help and inspiration through the years.

Contents

How to Dispose of this Book

Do me a favor...

Let me begin by making a request: If this life altering approach to weight loss turns out not to be for you, please dispose of it properly. Rather than simply putting it on a shelf with all of the other weight loss books that you may have collected, try find a good use for it—maybe stick it under the leg of a wobbly table, or use it to prop open a door. Or, perhaps it would make good tinder to start a fire in the winter, but I dread the thought of it being lumped in with all of the other useless "diet" books, written to make a quick buck for the author while taking advantage of the desperation of the obese. I hate the thought of it gathering dust waiting to be "read", packed and unpacked into a box during moves, and winding up being carried through life as useless baggage waiting for a better day.

By using this system of life management, I have lost over 100 pounds of fat, I have kept it off for over 20 years, and I have radically changed virtually every aspect of my life. The ideas presented here have completely altered my approach to living, and I feel that they are much too valuable to be dismissed as yet another "diet" book.

When I was fat, it never seemed odd to me that I was collecting diet books. I even kept them together on a special shelf, more than willing to tell anyone the good points of each. The books tended to take on a magical significance. They were a symbol of my good intentions—even though I don't think that I ever finished reading any of them. They all had the formula for success that I was desperately seeking, and as soon as the holidays (or whatever) were over, I was going to get serious about using one of them to do something about my problem.

It is very human to *intend* to do great things. We all want to make improvements in our lives but then we mysteriously set our intentions aside until we are in the mood, which never quite seems to happen.

I am not suggesting that everyone will be willing to try the concepts that I have included here. I am only asking that if you reach a point that you realize you no longer are willing to pursue this approach, that you be honest about that with yourself. I ask that you make a conscious decision to try this or not, but to be absolutely clear about it. So burn it, bury it, recycle it, or better yet read it. If I can convince you to do that, I feel that I will have accomplished something—and you will have too. Because even if your decision is that these ideas are not for you, you will have made a decision and acted upon it. And for a lot of people struggling with fat, that in itself is a tremendous accomplishment.

Who Am I?

I was a fat child who turned into an even fatter adult, frustrated and miserable. However, by using these techniques, I was able to transform myself from a fat blob on the couch watching television, to someone physically fit enough to run the 26.2 miles of the New York City Marathon.

I have no medical degree or training in psychology. For many years, I have felt that I wasn't an expert. I thought that there were many others who knew more and could do a much better job of explaining the things that I have found to be true, but I have come to question that. By reflecting on my own experiences—the doctors who never understood, the endless diet programs and books I've seen designed by "experts"—I have realized that I have a story worth telling. And it is a story that will be difficult for many to comprehend.

Others have occasionally looked at me with wonder, as if I've just stepped off a space ship from another planet. I have yet to meet a doctor who wasn't completely shocked when learning of my history. Even though the medical profession is devoted to helping people with their health, it has never been able to offer any lasting solution for weight loss. As a last resort, many have now turned to gastric bypass operations to treat obesity surgically, but I have read of some cases where even after such drastic measures the patient manages to regain weight. Surgery does not treat the real problem.

I'm quite sure that there is nothing special about me. I believe that anyone who is truly serious about dealing with compulsive overeating, and who uses this approach to life management, will experience results similar to mine.

The sad truth is that this book is not for everyone. Only a tiny percentage of the population ever manages to solve a weight problem, probably less than 5%.

Occasionally, when speaking to groups of fat people, I have become discouraged. Originally, I had fantasies of solving the entire world's fat problems by teaching these techniques. However, I quickly became frustrated when I found much of the audience still looking for a quick, painless fix. Many were not interested in learning life-changing concepts and were only looking for a simple solution to a very complex problem. I was ready to give up trying to teach what I've learned.

But then I had a realization: What if I had a cure for cancer, or AIDS, or any other terrible disease, that worked in 5% of the cases? Wouldn't a 5% success rate be enough to continue? Of course it would. In every group of fat people that I've spoken to, there are at least a few people with a glimmer of understanding in their eyes. After every class, there are always some who contact me to tell me of their successes and who have moved onto an entirely different path in life.

There are a tremendous number of people suffering from obesity. Certainly many of them are ready to get a handle on things, even if it means finally making genuine changes in their lives. Because, if they truly are in tune with themselves, they will know that that is exactly the problem—their lives, not their fat. It is about how they live and think about life, not how they look or what size clothing they wear. There can be no quick answer.

So first the bad news: *No weight loss program ever works (or ever will)*, and that includes this one. How could it? They are all just a collection of ideas. Some may be better than others, but all are only words printed on a page, and can do nothing unless put into action by the person reading them. There is no magic.

But now the good news: *Some of the people reading this will actually be willing to make significant improvements in their lives by applying these techniques.* They will be able to apply these concepts to radically change the quality of their lives, to accomplish things they never thought could be possible, and to lead a life that they've only dreamt about. And, that very likely could be you, if you are ready to seriously think about life in a new way, and genuinely address your fat problem.

I will attempt to be brutally honest, because that is the only way to begin to attack this problem. I will apologize in advance for what may sound like pessimism; I promise you that it is not. It is only that our culture is so full denial that anything that speaks the truth seems negative and unappealing. For example, politicians know this. They are rarely able to speak honestly, because they know that we don't want to hear the truth, and that we wouldn't elect them if we did. But I am not running for office. This is only for those who are ready to hear it.

And maybe even those that choose not to try this concept will benefit in some way, if only to stop the endless self-degradation of dieting and denial. By beginning to accept themselves as they are, they may just accomplish more than they realize.

What Is This?

This book is based on the ideas of Dr. Burt Bradley, a psychologist and radio talk show host. His original concept was surprisingly successful when used to combat smoking addictions, but I have found it to be every bit as powerful when managing compulsive overeating.

The method is built around four "cornerstones" that ultimately become the infrastructure for a healthier life. By coupling the Cornerstones with the notion of a paradigm shift, people are able to remake themselves into whomever they desire.

A food addiction is especially difficult to manage because there can be no "cold turkey" approach. The rules say you must eat or you will die. Smokers, alcoholics, or drug addicts can attack their dysfunctional behavior and be somewhat successful. If they are strong enough, they are able to completely remove it from their lifestyle. However, an overeater can never stop eating altogether. Imagine a smoker trying to limit himself to having only three cigarettes a day!

The need for food is at the core of the incredibly high failure rate when dealing with fat. A diet may *temporarily* control the eating disorder, but the inner turmoil will eventually drive the individual back to abusive eating. For anybody with an eating compulsion, any approach that does not deal with the whole person is doomed to failure.

This approach is not a diet, or a weight loss program. It is a system of life management that will build up the quality of life, making it possible to have a genuinely fulfilling life. As a by-product, it will produce weight loss, but that is not really its purpose.

This is a methodology, not a program. It is something that does not have an end. It is a way of living. It contains the tools to have *whatever you want* in life, to become whoever you want to be. For me, that started with wanting to lose a lot of fat, but it has gone much further. Furthermore, I expect it to continue until the last day of my life, producing ongoing benefits—many of which have absolutely nothing to do with being thin.

These are behavioral techniques. They are based in action, not analysis. However, many deep insights become apparent as new behaviors are adopted and the underlying problems are flushed out into the open.

This book describes the techniques that I use, and my experiences and views of Dr. Bradley's original concepts. It also includes much that I have learned and added to his basic ideas. We do not always agree, and I suspect that anyone reading this will not always agree with me either. This approach is very much a personal journey, and will not be identical for any two people. However, the basic tenets are sound and apply to everyone. The book that you are holding in your hands is a complete guide to these state-of-the-art techniques, powerful enough to permanently correct your eating disorder—if you are truly ready.

Introduction

Pre-Cornerstone Experiences

I was always fat, or at least it seems that way. I felt fat and behaved fat. It is odd now to look back at childhood pictures. I really wasn't a grossly fat kid early on, but somehow that idea found its way into my identity and became a self-fulfilling prophecy. I remember hearing the traditional euphemisms, "heavy", "husky", "big-boned" etc., but I picked up on the idea of being fat, no matter what anyone called it.

As my parents pushed to get me active, it served instead to reinforce the whole notion that I was inactive. I spent hours watching television and fantasizing about being someone else. I thwarted every effort my parents came up with to restrict my eating. I could always find food and took pride in outwitting them. It became a game. In the process, I came to view myself as fat and worthless and developed a genuinely serious weight problem.

As I got older, the fat itself became the problem. It was my identity. I was not athletic or very coordinated as boys were supposed to be—additional proof of my worthlessness—and more reason to withdraw into my own comfortable fat world. It was who I was. And, it felt *so good* to eat. It was my main source of real pleasure.

As I moved into my teenage years and realized what the implications of being fat would be when it came to attracting girls, the problem became harder to ignore. First, I developed that wonderful human skill of denial. Just rearrange the facts so that the problem no longer existed in my mind.

I would rarely have my photograph taken, for example, because with a picture there could be no denying what I looked like. Photographs didn't lie, so I did my best to make sure they didn't exist. When there was a camera around, I wasn't.

I wore clothes that I thought hid the problem—baggy clothes with vertical stripes that made me look thinner, or so I thought. I learned to look in the mirror and see something that wasn't there, or should I say, not see something that was there. I would suck in my stomach and position myself in a way that a more flattering view would appear.

If I ever climbed onto a scale, I learned to shift my weight around and flap my arms to manipulate the scale's reading to a more acceptable weight. And if all else failed, I would simply pretend that I wasn't as fat as I was.

Buying clothes was always the worst. There was no avoiding knowing my clothing size, and it would provide unavoidable proof that I was fat. I remember being measured for a tuxedo for senior prom in high school. When the salesman asked me what size pants I thought I would need, I told him size 34. I had convinced myself that I actually wore a size 34 pants. He looked at me with disbelief as he put the tape measure around me and read out a 46 inch waist. I remember wishing that a hole would open beneath me, a very large hole, and that I could disappear into it. For years whenever I'd see the photographs taken at that prom, I would curse that salesman for sizing me in such a huge tux that made me look like a blimp. I could always rearrange the facts anyway that I needed to avoid reality.

It is odd how I was able to see the fat as a separate issue. It was something that really had nothing to do with me personally. I thought it would be great to just get it cut off, then I'd be fine, and my life would be great.

I despised that fat so much. It was like a big cloud of lard that surrounded me at all times. Underneath, I felt that I was a good person. The fat part was the bad part. If I could just dispose of it, all of my self-loathing would go with it.

Eventually, I discovered the deadly world of dieting. It had all of the components I was looking for. I believed that the right diet would magically melt the pounds off quickly, and once that was over, I could be happy and popular and have a wonderful life. I just had to endure the diet for a while and everything would be fixed.

Diets had an additional plus—you could plan when you'd start one. You could pick a future date to begin and feel better because you were *planning* to do something about the problem, all the time looking forward to some wonderful future time when life would be great. Diets were like pre-packaged denial. I could calculate what date I wanted to be thin and work backwards from there to determine when to start the diet. There was no sense in doing it any sooner than that. Dieting had taught me another useful skill—living in the future. Oh, the great things I was going to do once I got rid of that fat! But somehow, I never quite did.

I tried every diet that came along. I bought every diet book, joined Weight Watchers and their competitors over and over. I was always looking for the magic solution.

Every diet began with the obligatory weight chart. You'd look up your height, decide whether you had a large, medium, or small frame (large of course), and there would be the *correct* weight: Your goal—that point at which life would begin.

Next came **THE DIET**. The fix. Eat this. Drink this. Don't eat that. And poof! Problem solved. It didn't matter what kind of diet it was, the message was always the same—"This is where you belong and how you must behave to get there."

And the diets *worked*. I'd start with the rush of excitement that *this* was going to be it. I couldn't wait to get through it and get my life going. Of course, I'd have to carry around Tupperware containers full of whatever it was I was supposed to be eating on **THE DIET**. I'd have to skip parties or pass on dinner invitations for a while, because they wouldn't be "legal", but it was worth it. Shortly, I'd be normal. I'd fit in and I'd belong.

The results were always the same. The diet worked—I just didn't. I'd usually manage to lose about 30 of the 100+ pounds that I needed to lose and then just run out of steam, collapsing in self-disgust. I would spend all kinds of money to find out what *normal* was, to be given the *solution*, and all I had to do was follow it. But I couldn't do even that simple thing. *They* had the answer, but *I* couldn't do it. **THE DIET** was worthwhile; I was worthless. I was anything but normal. I wasn't worthy of anything. I had no willpower—that mystical power that everyone else seemed to have.

So I'd always quit **THE DIET**. Maybe the holidays would be coming so I'd decide to wait for them to be over. Then I'd start over again so I could solve the problem before the summer swimsuit season came. But summer would come and I hadn't done much. Maybe the fall would be better. So I'd start again in September with back-to-school enthusiasm. But the holidays would be coming and it would be better to wait until they were over to *really* start…

Years passed but the pattern never changed. My life just dragged on with a lot of dull, throbbing pain. I was one of the brightest in my class in college. I had a 4.00 grade point average in a high demand field, but few companies were interested in hiring me. The rejection letters came with the usual non-explanatory "we really enjoyed talking with you, however...". But I didn't need an explanation, I knew the true reason for the rejection: fat. It didn't matter what I could do or how bright I was. It did matter what I looked like. I was a walking advertisement of my lack of self-control. I couldn't even follow a simple diet. I wasn't normal, how could I possibly be a good employee? I didn't fault their reasoning, I *agreed* with it. All I had to do was just eat what I was supposed to—so simple—and I couldn't do it. I didn't deserve a good job. I didn't deserve any recognition. Not until I could get myself together.

I felt I deserved nothing. I'd buy the cheapest clothes at the discount stores, clip-on ties, polyester suits—the bare minimum to get by. I wasn't worth spending any money on, at least not until I deserved it. There was no point in investing in myself until I lost the weight, which I was always just about ready to do.

Fortunately, I did manage to find a job, not the one I had dreamt about, but one that I could at least work at quietly and go unnoticed (until I could lose the weight and get my life started).

I would starve off the weight, losing hundreds of pounds over the years, but I was still me. The fat was always there mentally, if not physically, and I'd always quickly gain it back. I was still somebody who ate too much. I might be able occasionally to impose some behavioral restrictions on myself, but only temporarily. I hoped that life would be wonderful once I lost the fat, but it never really would change, and I'd go right back to who I *really* was, gaining all of the weight back, and usually a few more pounds than I'd started with.

I was almost 30 years old when I stumbled across a class taught by Dr. Bradley called *The Psychology of Losing Weight and Never Finding It Again*. He taught us about four "cornerstones" that finally gave me the tools that I needed to start truly creating the life that I sought.

Fortunately, by the time I took his class I think I had finally exhausted my desire for the quick fix. At some level, I was beginning to see that what I had tried for years wasn't going to get me what I wanted. It seems silly now, looking back. Why couldn't I have seen that what I was doing was causing more problems and solving nothing? For some reason, I was incapable of seeing that. Dr. Bradley's ideas allowed me to change every aspect of my life completely, and I will forever be indebted to him.

There has always been a part of me that knows that so many more people are suffering every bit as much as I was, and I feel a duty to give his ideas a wider exposure. So, I have written my interpretations of his ideas and added my own experiences to further define the process. The book is constructed to be interactive so that you can begin to implement the concepts in your own life.

Dr. Bradley has frequently included me as a guest speaker at his course, and I have related many of these stories. Surprisingly, even after all of these years, some of the experiences were so painful that they are still quite difficult to recount. However, I'll do my best to describe the transformation that I have experienced, and to do it in a way that will be of value to the reader.

I believe that this book will be useful to anyone who reads it and is truly ready for the concepts presented. I feel that even a "thin" person could benefit tremendously from this approach to living, and in fact that is the basic idea. This is the way a "well" person lives. It has nothing to do with being fat or thin. It has to do with being alive and well.

1

Paradigms

A paradigm is a way of looking at things. Like a pair of eyeglasses, it alters what we see and affects our interpretation of life. We all see life through our own paradigms, and for the most part, are completely unaware of their existence.

What I never understood when I was fat was that I saw life through a "fat" paradigm. Being fat was fundamental to my identity and to my understanding of how life worked. Consciously I could think about being somebody else, but unconsciously I *knew* better. The diets weren't *really* going to work. I wasn't *really* going to change. Fat people are fat just like tall people are tall and short people are short. Nobody goes on tall diets, do they?

To begin understanding the Cornerstone process, I think it is worthwhile first to look at the concept of a paradigm and a paradigm shift and to begin to see ourselves from a more objective and detached point of view. Before beginning any journey, it is important to develop a realistic idea of just where we want to be heading.

Paradigm Shifts

Our minds are full of paradigms so that we can interpret what happens to us and around us. Paradigms are such powerful belief systems that we rarely are aware that they even exist. Sometimes the paradigms are useful, and sometimes they need to give way to new information. When this new belief system takes hold, it is referred to as a paradigm shift. A new paradigm must be constructed to takes the place of the original one.

I first learned of the paradigm concept from Stephen Covey's book *The Seven Habits of Highly Effective People*. He gives an example of riding on a subway and being annoyed by a fellow passenger's children who are running around the car disturbing people. The children's father ignores the situation and allows his children to continue annoying the other passengers. Finally, Covey is irritated enough to ask the father why he doesn't control his children. The father replies, "Oh, you're right. I guess I should do something about it. We just came from the hospital where their mother died about an hour ago. I don't know what to think and I guess they don't know how to handle it either."

This example shows how in an instant an entirely new view of the same situation can take place. The original paradigm classified the father and children as merely annoying and inconsiderate. The new paradigm had to incorporate the reasons for the children's misbehavior and bring an entirely new set of interpretations. When new information was introduced that contradicted the original assumptions, a new set of rules emerged and changed altered the frame of reference.

That was the first I'd heard of either a paradigm or a paradigm shift. I realized that a paradigm shift might also be used to describe the internal change that occurred within me years before allowing me to redefine myself.

Until I learned about this approach to life, I never truly believed that a fat person could genuinely do something about obesity. Fat people go on diets and then they go off diets. They certainly aren't physically active, and even if they manage to lose a few pounds, they will always gain them back. That was my old paradigm.

In its strictest sense a paradigm is a model of something, a collection of rules that explain how something functions. However, the term has come to mean a model of our thoughts, a way of thinking about things that represents our personal belief systems. We all have internal maps and rules defining how the world works. For example, we know that if we drop a ball, it will fall to the ground. That could be called the gravity paradigm. But, if you were an astronaut in a weightless environment on the space shuttle, you would quickly find that you were now in a new paradigm. If you drop a ball, it would probably just hang in space, maybe even drift away. That would be a paradigm shift. The rules, which used to be immutable, have now changed completely. All bets are off.

The concept of a paradigm isn't difficult to understand, but understanding or even being aware of our personal paradigms is all but impossible. Our belief

systems are so powerful that we don't even see them as beliefs. They are virtually invisible to us. Our experiences are our frame of reference for everything
else that happens. It is how we make sense of the chaos that surrounds us. It is
a sort of internal filing system that allows us to continue living our lives without having to analyze every moment.

Many components of a paradigm probably are true, but they are never
absolute. In a different setting, as in the Space Shuttle example, perfectly valid
rules become perfectly invalid. When we encounter something that doesn't fit
our paradigm we usually do our best to ignore it, and when we can't, we have a
paradigm shift.

A good analogy often used to describe a paradigm is that of a map. The
map tells you where you are, what to expect around the corner, and what
choices are available. If you follow it, the outcome is quite predictable and
everything will work out—but only if you are in the right city.

Now, take that map and try to use it in a different city and you will quickly
get into trouble. It won't matter how diligently you follow it or how carefully
you plan your trip, you won't get to the right place. If the map provides any
value at all, it would be a coincidence.

Dieting is really a paradigm, a supposed map out of fat city; a map that
everybody accepts as gospel. However, the strange thing about dieting is that
it never works, at least not in the sense that the fat is lost and never comes
back. Fat people using the diet paradigm frequently give credit to the diet and
blame themselves for not losing the fat or not keeping it off. It is rare to hear
anyone suggest that the diet map isn't going to work. It never seems to matter
how diligently dieters follow the program or how careful they are about the
instructions. Ultimately, it doesn't work (and I define working as a *permanent
and lasting weight loss*) and the dieters blame themselves.

The Two Category Fat Paradigm

Being fat is itself a paradigm. Being fat brings with it a whole set of assumptions—assumptions that usually the fat person and the rest of the world accept
without question.

Possibly the deadliest aspect of the fat paradigm is that it creates a warped
perspective of life. The world appears divided into simple categories—the "fat"
and the "un-fat". The "fat" are miserable and the "un-fat" are not, or so it
seems. The distortion occurs because the fat people experience so little *because*
of their fat. It is their barrier and their comfort. The world of the un-fat is seen

13

unattainable, like the glamorous world of movie
1 unavailable. Most of us assume that a movie star could
and we are always shocked when the details of their trou-
the tabloids as if it is some strange and rare occurrence.
es the same illusion. If only we were thin, we would have no
more problem. Our fat is the focal point of all of our frustrations. When I'd
begin a diet, I'd feel like I was finally getting an opportunity to cross through
the great fat barrier. But, as I moved through it, I would feel quite vulnerable.
Not only were my problems not disappearing they were usually bothering me
more. My fat insulation was being stripped away exposing me to all of the
things that I was hiding from. My life was not improving by leaps and bounds.

To make matters worse, people would start to notice me. It was flattering
but frightening and nothing that I had any experience with. My old problems
weren't solved and I was being flooded with new problems that I was even less
equipped to handle.

The premise of all diets is that life will be so wonderful once the goal
weight is attained that the dieter will be motivated to maintain the weight.
Nothing could be more wrong. Now that I can look back at my dieting experiences objectively, I can see the flaws in the diet paradigm that I was using. I
can see clearly that my failures came from the fact that I was learning nothing
about coping with life which had been the real problem all along. In fact, the
diet was stripping away my only coping mechanism—food.

I was always convinced that the *diet* worked and *I* failed. Try an experiment: Ask any fat person if they've had any experiences with diets that work.
Virtually all of them will begin a dissertation of the various "successes" that
they have had with diets. Even though you will be talking with a fat person,
they will inevitably be labeling the diets as successful and implicitly labeling
themselves as failures. These are the signs of the diet paradigm and the fat
paradigm at work.

The idea of losing weight really represents a paradigm itself. It conjures up
images of cottage cheese, carrot sticks, bulging sweat pants, grueling exercise
regimes, and aching muscles. In general, it represents a program of self-depri-
vation and punishment. It has a definite beginning (usually a Monday that has
been preceded by a "last supper" of incredible indulgence). And, it has a definite end, usually in the form of a "goal weight", some point when all of this
torture will end and we can get back to life which will now be wonderful.
Almost nobody ever makes it to the end so rarely is that last assumption of the
paradigm challenged with reality.

The very term "losing weight" is nonsense. Nobody that I know of cares how much they weigh, they care how fat they are. Why doesn't anybody say "losing fat"? And for that matter, nobody really cares how fat they are, they just want to look good. They want people to respond to them with more love or respect and maybe feel a little bit healthier in the process. We've tied our self-image to the scale simply because we can measure our weight much easier than we could measure what it is that we really seek.

We torture ourselves with this dieting stuff, and then go right back to the way things were—the good old fat paradigm—which is no surprise to anybody. It is as if we must do this periodically to prove that we really do care about ourselves and have the best of intentions, but we just can't quite make it. Underneath all of that blubber, we are good people.

Nobody "loses weight". It virtually never happens yet we all seem to believe that it does. Every time I see a new doctor for one reason or another and I recount my fat history, the reaction is always one of genuine shock followed by questions about "how I did it". The *doctor* is asking *me* how *I* did it. The trained health professional don't know how to get people to improve their lives, yet they go on prescribing diets to their fat patients with neither doctors nor the patients truly believing that it will do any lasting good at all.

The important point here that must be understood is that dieting is a paradigm, not a paradigm shift. Being fat is a paradigm, and being un-fat is a paradigm.

To illustrate this point, picture a very attractive thin person (one you secretly hate and would love to do something mean to). Let's call her Cyndi. She is one of those gorgeous people that seem able to eat whatever they want whenever they want; she is a perky, bouncy, pretty person who has life under control and spends no time at all worrying about her weight. How could you not hate somebody like that?

Now, picture yourself with an evil, black magic fat spell. The spell creates an instantaneous reverse diet that piles on 100 pounds of fat instantly. One night, you sneak into Cyndi's bedroom and secretly cast the fat spell so that the next morning she wakes up and is now **FAT.** You chuckle to yourself the next day as you watch her desperately trying to find clothes that fit and that hide all of that hideous fat. No more skin tight jeans for Cyndi.

However, what do you think would happen to Cyndi long term? Would she start overeating simply because she was fat? Would she make sure that she consumed tremendous amounts of calories to maintain her fat? I doubt it. Chances are she would continue, as best she could, with the lifestyle that she led before becoming fat. And, after enough time, she would be right back were she started—thin. Cyndi wouldn't be able to maintain her fat anymore than a fat person can maintain a diet.

In a diet (or as in the fictitious example, reverse diet) the individual's paradigm *has not shifted*. A temporary condition is imposed but the basic belief system *remains completely intact*. Could any other long-term results really be expected?

To solve a problem with obesity, we must create a paradigm shift, not merely modify our behavior. We must change our entire point of reference and belief system.

My Fat Paradigm Shift

For me, I think the turning point came somewhat trivially and months before I actually took Dr. Bradley's class. One day at work, I accidentally spilled coffee on my shirt. It was one of those cheap, polyester shirts that I used to wear when I was fat. My paradigm stated that a fat person didn't deserve quality clothing.

The problem was that the stain was horribly obvious against the background of the white shirt. As a fat person, I felt that the worst possible thing was to draw attention to myself. I was frantic and horribly embarrassed. I avoided people as much as possible to hide the stain. Then, at lunchtime, I went to a nearby department store to buy a new shirt to wear the rest of the day. Unfortunately, I was working downtown and there were no K-Marts or discounts stores nearby. My only choice was to go to an upscale department store that offered only expensive shirts.

I can remember standing there trying to decide what to do. The shirts they sold were easily three times as expensive as the ones that I wore. I felt as if I didn't deserve even to be in such a store let alone getting ready to purchase something. Nevertheless, the thought of being noticed and looking like a slob for the rest of the day induced me to buy my first quality shirt. Moreover, I decided I'd better get one that fit comfortably now, rather than one that I could "get into" after I started losing weight (another dieter's "trick"). With the price as high as it was, I was going to need to wear it a long time.

I think in that instant, and possibly for the first time, I was brutally honest with myself. I had no immediate plans to start a diet, so I bought a shirt that fit. I remember being struck by the fact that they actually had shirts in my size—that somebody thought that someone as fat as I was could be worthy of such quality. I bought it and put it on in the restroom. I ran my hands down the sleeves and felt the quality of the cloth. I could button the collar comfortably. I can still remember finding every excuse to look at that shirt the rest of the day. It was as if a subtle realization had occurred—I was worthwhile just like I was. The shirt proved it. I didn't have to be thin to feel worthwhile: a **paradigm shift**.

I went back the next day and bought several more along with some expensive ties. Somehow, I'd decided that I was worth it. In its small way, my coffee stain had destroyed my notion of the fat and the un-fat, the worthy and the unworthy. It had let me stand outside my paradigm and see it for what it was—an invalid set of assumptions.

That day a small event had set something in motion that would ultimately result in huge changes. Not by itself, but it caused me to rethink my self-image and made me receptive to some new ideas that I probably would have ignored before. The stage was set for a new paradigm.

The Grief Cycle

When a belief system dies, and before a new one can take its place, we typically experience the *grief cycle*. This is the same set of emotions that a grieving person experiences after the death of a loved one, but they occur in other situations as well. The stages are:

- Denial
- Anger
- Bargaining
- Depression
- Acceptance

Although the grief cycle typically is associated with an actual death, I've found that it comes into play anytime we let go of something like then end of a relationship or even a set of beliefs.

I had an opportunity to watch the grief cycle in action with my youngest daughter. Children seem able to process new ideas more quickly, perhaps because they have less invested in the old ones, but even so they still experience the grief cycle and they can give us an opportunity to observe it in a relatively short period of time.

My youngest daughter has always had a vivid imagination. Because of this, she was able to accept the idea of Santa Claus much longer than other children of her age. Whatever new information she would encounter that contradicted her beliefs could be ignored or re-cataloged in some way that supported her belief. Certainly, every Christmas would bring tangible evidence that Santa Claus was real. Still, from somewhere deep inside of her would come nagging doubts. As she grew older, her experience with the rest of life began to challenge her belief system.

One day I took her to a museum that was featuring an exhibit of children's illustrators over the last 100 years. Many of the books contained drawings of Santa Claus, but they looked very different from the drawings of today. Even his name varied over the years before settling on today's name and image.

This obviously bothered her. She seemed deep in thought all of the way home from the museum. This wasn't just her older sister tormenting her with contradictions. This wasn't a fellow classmate taunting her with an opposing view. It was tangible, unbiased evidence from the past that Santa wasn't always quite like he is today. And if that were true, couldn't it be possible that he really wasn't real at all?

Finally, after we returned home, she pinned me down for specifics. Was Santa Claus real? Not wanting to shatter her, I tried the "Yes, Virginia" approach. Santa was real, I said, as long as you believed in him. That wasn't going to work this time. She wanted the facts. I could sense her anger growing as she moved out of denial, so I mustered up my courage and tried gently to tell her the truth.

Her paradigm let go with an explosion. All at once denial was over and anger was in control. She flew out of the room with a wail, screaming all of the way up the stairs before slamming her bedroom door. She had been deceived by life, her parents and herself, and she was angry.

I shuddered with guilt. How could I have spared her this pain? About 20 minutes later she returned, this time weeping with the anger gone but bargaining now in control. "The Easter Bunny is real though, isn't he?" she asked.

There was no turning back, as I once again confessed the truth. Again, she moved from denial, this time for the Easter Bunny paradigm, flew into a rage and ran back upstairs.

Twenty more minutes passed and then finally the anger turned to tears and sobs. Depression. Sadness. After a little more time, she returned. Exhausted, but calm, and with a slightly more mature look in her eyes. Acceptance. In fact, she seemed almost happy. She had processed the new information, moved into a new paradigm, and all of the sudden she felt more grownup. She was now part of a new group of older non-believers. It felt right to her. The nagging doubts were gone, she was a little more mature, and that was something that she truly wanted more than the belief in Santa.

Think about the grief cycle in terms of being fat. Initially, we try our best to deny or reduce the problem in our minds—denial. Baggy clothes, swimming suits that cover everything, or a T-shirt worn over a swimsuit to "reduce sunburn", avoiding being photographed, sucking our stomachs in while looking in the mirror, flapping our arms when on the scale, planning a new diet that we're going to start "on Monday", deciding that we're "big boned" instead of fat. There is no end to the creativity of the human mind.

But finally, usually through some event that we can't deny, we decide to try to do something about the problem. Maybe even our "loosest" piece of clothing refuses to fit anymore. Maybe the scale finally moves into new territory. Maybe a doctor scares us during a physical. Possibly some event like a wedding or a class reunion forces us to try to attack the problem. So we begin **THE DIET**. We take this *thing*, whatever the latest, greatest craze is, and we apply *it* to ourselves.

Monday we start. We begin with great hope and anticipation. Whatever diet we are using however, is anything but natural to our way of life. We think we can do this for a while, but we are quite sure that we want it over quickly. Is it any wonder that the all of the diet programs promise some sort of *quick* results? Sure, we're eager to be gorgeous, but we're also eager to get through this hell and the diet marketers know it. So, if you want to sell your diet, you talk about how quickly it will work because everybody knows they won't be able to endure it for long.

Depending on the severity of **THE DIET**, we start to experience the next phase—anger. We get very grumpy. We miss our fat food. How could we not? What prepared us for this harsh change in lifestyle? We might blame it on the food (or lack of food) that we are consuming. Maybe it is sugar or fat withdrawals. However, most people will find themselves feeling quite upset in one form or another. We may be losing weight, but not fast enough. Now all that seems to remain is never-ending torture.

At this point, we begin to move into bargaining—or cheating as it might be called in dieting parlance—anything to cope with the misery. A little more food than **THE DIET** calls for or maybe some foods that it doesn't. Can frozen yogurt really be fattening? Certainly not if you eat it right out of the car-ton. Do I really need to eat *all* of that broiled fish? Wouldn't deep-fried be close enough? How about just one peanut? (The only time I ever managed to eat just one peanut was when I found one under the couch cushions.) I can't just throw away all of the food that the kids don't eat. I've got to go to this lunch/dinner/party, so I'll just suspend **THE DIET** for now. I'll go ahead and temporarily slip off this diet and make up for it tomorrow. Maybe this just wasn't the week to get started on a diet, there is so much going on right now. I'll start again next week, that should produce better results. And besides, I just heard about a *better* diet that I think I'll try. There is no limit to the excuses.

The vast, vast majority of dieters give up after the bargaining phase. The attempt to modify behavior has finished and the return to denial is much more appealing. What else could be expected? With the death of a loved one, there can be no turning back. But with dieting, it is still the option of the dieter to put things back the way they were. So much for grieving.

A small percentage of dieters drive themselves forward through pure deter-mination to the next phase—depression. They are going to make it, by God, and they do. Sort of.

Maybe the complements of friends have been enough to keep the dieter moving forward. The flirtatious looks from strangers that have never hap-pened before, the new wardrobe, whatever new thrills it takes to supplant the addiction and to survive the inner pain of grief.

But, at some point, the outside world adjusts to the thinner person and it takes less and less notice of the dieter. The thrills begin to fade and the old inner self is still in there, begging to return. A wave of sadness begins to wash over the dieter like the tide returning.

Although most of my early dieting attempts ended in the bargaining phase, twice I managed to drive myself all the way to my "goal weight". The sadness was unbearable. Eventually, nobody noticed that I was thin and I didn't know who I was anymore. I used to carry a fat picture in my wallet and pull it out to show people how fat I "used" to be. I didn't realize it, but I was trying to find the thrill of having somebody complement me, as a way of lifting myself out of the depression.

In the "thin" world, nothing works the same. Strangers notice you when in the past they ignored you. Think about how instinctively you move away from a fat person standing in the aisle at the grocery store, or in an elevator. I used to be unaware that the seat next to me on the subway would be one of the last taken as the train filled with people. Now, people sat *next* to me—by choice—long before it was the only remaining seat. People would brush against me in an elevator, crowd into me at a store, start conversations with me for no apparent reason.

Women in particular have a difficult time. Men start "hitting" on them. Sound wonderful? To the inexperienced, it is terribly frightening. Fat people are used to being invisible. Now they are exposed and vulnerable with no idea how to proceed.

If that weren't enough, the people that have known us all along begin to resent us. Maybe a spouse is jealous of the attention, real or imagined. Maybe fat friends resent our determination and success. Maybe they miss the trips to the favorite restaurant, or the snacks enjoyed together in front of the television. We have inadvertently sent the people around us into their own grief cycle and it is unlikely that they are as willing to experience it as we are, and very likely will find unconscious ways to sabotage us.

Ideally, the dieter would only need to hang on long enough for the depression to lift and move on into the acceptance phase. An even smaller percentage of people manage that. In most cases, the new "thin" world is so terrifying and the depression so pervasive that the only way out is to bring back the fat barrier as rapidly as possible.

If *being* fat is bad, it is nothing compared to rapidly *regaining* fat. I once regained 10 pounds a month for a year after losing 80 pounds on a diet. I couldn't wear clothes more than a month without finding larger things to wear. Try as I might to stop eating, something inside of me was now in control. As a fat person, I used to pretend that my metabolism was somehow different, that I really was under control and just an unfortunate victim. Now I had no excuse. I had proven that my metabolism was fine. My weakness and lack of self-control was there for everybody to see, pound after pound. My self-worth plummeted to new lows. I could see the looks in people's eyes, "What are you doing, why are you getting so fat?" If there were any doubts before, they were gone. I truly despised myself.

Although most of this behavior is unconscious on the part of the dieter and the surrounding world, I believe that the sub-conscious is quite aware of it. It is busy cataloging the experience and modifying behavior patterns to be more defensive, to make sure this *never* happens again. Life was better before; forget what everybody has been telling you about losing weight. Is it any wonder that dieters regain all of their weight and then some? Could this extra fat possibly be an additional measure of security to prevent future suffering? Is it any wonder that each subsequent diet becomes harder and less effective?

Unwanted Paradigm Shifts

Frequently, a paradigm is shifted only as the result of a crisis. A smoker is told of a spot on his lung in a routine physical. An obese person has a mild heart attack. Someone who never thought about job security is laid off and forced into the job market. A marriage is rocked by an affair, or the death of a spouse. A parent dies and forces us to confront our own mortality.

Typically, it takes an external crisis to jar us out of a paradigm and make us realize that we really do have other choices, even if they are unwanted. It can require being brutally thrown outside our paradigm even to be able to see that we were ever in one.

What we want to accomplish here is to be able to recognize our current paradigm and then choose to change it before something changes it for us. It is much more desirable to decide to step outside the comfort of our current paradigm and begin work on a new one of our own choosing rather than wait for something else to choose for us.

Finding Your Current Fat Paradigm

To begin to make genuine changes you first must understand where you are right now. Read through the following list of common fat beliefs and check any that you have thought about yourself or fat people in general.

- Fat people need to go on a diet to correct the problem.

- Fat people have a slow metabolism.

- If I am fat, nobody will find me attractive.

- If I am thin, everybody will find me attractive.

- As we get older, we get fatter.

- If I could manage to lose weight, I will feel so good about myself that I won't gain it back.

- A scale is the appropriate measure of progress in losing weight.

- I don't eat any more or any worse than thin people, I'm just naturally fat.
- I've been fat all of my life, I was meant to be fat.
- I inherited my fat from my parents; it's in my genes.
- I have no self-control.
- Fat people are jolly.
- My real problem is that I am big boned.
- If I ever really lost weight, I would just gain it back.
- Muscle turns into fat if it's not used.
- I have more fat cells than thin people do.
- I'm fundamentally a fat person and different from a thin person.

Now add some of your own if you can. Try to think of things that maybe you *wish* weren't true, but tend to believe *are* true. Remember, the beliefs that define a paradigm may actually be true, but it is still important to be aware of your personal frame of reference.

- _____
- _____
- _____
- _____
- _____
- _____
- _____
- _____
- _____
- _____
- _____

Defining Your New Paradigm

In the previous section, did you select any of the choices? Did you actually circle or check the ones that applied to you, I mean actually pick up a pen, put it on the page and make a mark? How about any additional items, did you think of any? Did you actually *write down* what you thought? If you did, put your hand up in the air, reach back, and give yourself a big pat on the back. You are obviously serious about tackling your problem. If you didn't, don't be discouraged. What you are experiencing is a touch of denial. It is lurking inside you, just trying to steer you off course. Maybe you thought about the examples, even nodded your head in agreement, but you didn't actually do anything about it. That will spell trouble down the road, and as the old saying goes—the road to hell is paved with good intentions. Go back and really *do* the exercise. Pay attention to how it feels to have your intellect overrule your instincts. You may feel anger or disgust while you write. You may mutter to yourself about the silliness of actually needing to write, possibly cursing me in the process. If so, you are feeling the beginnings of a mini-grief cycle, denial being challenged by anger. Many people will not even take this tiny step toward changing their lives.

If you are seriously resisting writing on the page, you might want to stop now and re-read the section on disposing of this book! On the other hand, *don't give up* if you are still interested in solving your problem but just can't quite get yourself moving. This is all a radical change to your thinking and you might not be quite ready to deal with the changes yet. Keep reading and return to any of the exercises when you genuinely feel ready for them.

Once you've done the exercise, you should have at least some ideas about your current paradigm. Discovering your paradigm is a frustrating process. It is a little bit like feeling your way around a room that is completely dark, stumbling over some things and missing others completely. This process goes on for a long time. The best way to make a paradigm reveal itself is to begin to move outside of it and see what barriers you encounter. To continue with the dark room analogy, maybe you can see a stream of light coming from under a door on the other side of the room, or maybe there are several possible doors to choose from. On the other side of those doors, lies a new paradigm. It may be as simple as walking towards the light and opening the door and stepping through. But chances are it isn't or you would have done that a long time ago. Most likely there are unseen obstacles that you will trip over, stub your toe on, or that in some other way will frustrate your progress. You must feel your way slowly and carefully, stopping when you have to, rubbing your injured shins, maybe retracing steps if necessary, but never giving up. To give up is to sit in that dark room forever scared and lost. You must never lose sight of the direction that you are headed and be willing to accept what happens along the way if you want to make true progress.

Therefore, the next step is to get at least an initial idea of where you are headed, what direction in the dark room you wish to go, and towards which door you want to move. This is not nearly as easy as it sounds. Most of us have simply accepted that we shouldn't be fat and have never thought much beyond that. That idea is merely a part of our current paradigm, not a part of a new one. It is part of being fat to think that you shouldn't be; it comes with the package. Everybody thinks that fat people should lose weight.

What you must discover is *why you want to* lose weight, not why you should. "Should" has nothing to do with it. Other people's ideas have nothing to do with it. It must be yours and yours alone. It must represent what you truly desire or you will never get there.

What do you think would be different if you were thin? Most people will start with some initial talk about health concerns, but I don't think that we're all that concerned about health, even though we think we should be. Dig deeper, be brutally honest with yourself. What would be better? More respect? More affection? More love? What barriers does the fat represent?

I think that a good approach to finding your new paradigm is to find some time by yourself, lie down, close your eyes, and relax. Picture yourself now, how you look, what you do with your time, and with whom you interact regularly. Then gently switch your mind to a new channel. It will probably be poor reception at first, but keep watching and see what appears. What would you be if you had no barriers? What would you *really* look like? Losing fat does not necessarily mean becoming gorgeous; there are plenty of thin people who aren't attractive. Once I lost my fat I was shocked to find out that I was short. I know that sounds ridiculous, but being fat was so overriding in my self-image I never even considered how tall I was. Being a short man is definitely a handicap in our culture, so it wasn't that my appearance problems melted away with the pounds.

Be honest with yourself. Picture yourself *doing* new things—things that are appealing to you. Don't just imagine yourself looking better. How would you spend your time? Who would you spend it with? What kind of people would you like to associate with?

For many, even calling up these fantasies brings tremendous guilt. It might mean that we have to admit to ourselves that some people that are close to us wouldn't be part of this new picture; they wouldn't get roles in our new script. But this script is not finished nor completely cast, so continue with the fantasy and don't worry about the all of the details, you can and will continue to change it as you go along. This is for you right now. Assume no barriers, no responsibilities, and no guilt. What would your life be like if you could have any wishes granted?

If your new script contains descriptions like "I would be very wealthy", you need to dig deeper. What would you do with that money? How would you spend your time? The world is full of rich, miserable people. Are you really wishing to be free of some particular burden, maybe a dependency on someone else, or a job that you aren't satisfied with? Money is a lot like fat. It is a stand-in for other issues and tends to mask what we really want or don't want.

Also, don't forget that you may be already living the life that you want. There is no law that says you must be thin to be happy. Maybe eating is such a pleasure that there could be no new life that would equal the happiness you already have. Maybe all that you need is the courage to face the world and be happy with yourself as you are right now.

Some Things Worth Doing

I remember tucking one of my daughters into bed one night, when she was about 3 or 4 years old. She was talking about what she wanted to be when she grew up. Then she switched subjects and asked me what I had wanted to be when I was a kid. I told her that I'd wanted to be a musician. She looked at me with innocent eyes and asked, "Well, is that what you are?"

In that simple moment I'd realized how I'd lost track of something that was important to me. Music. To a young child, it's as simple as wanting and then being. To an adult it is complicated and unattainable. Or is it? Where do we learn that lesson? What is it about responsibility that makes us think we can't do what we want? I'd been so busy working, paying bills, planning for retirement, maintaining my life, that I'd missed some very important aspects of what I was trying to do in the first place. Shortly after that moment with my daughter, I bought a piano and began teaching myself to play. It was tremendously rewarding and it had nothing to do with being fat or thin.

Try to think of three things that you would do if you were who you wanted to be. Write them down. If they are too embarrassing to write in this book, write them on a separate sheet of paper and then destroy it if you are worried about another person reading it. But do *write it down*. Don't just think about it. As I will say repeatedly in this book, the power is in the writing not the reading or the thinking. Writing forces your brain to use different processes and will have profound effects on your behavior. Trust me on that.

Don't worry if you can't imagine yourself *really* doing these things, the purpose of this is simply to get an idea about which direction you would like to go as opposed to where you are right now. If you always wanted to be an astronaut, put it down. If you always wanted to attend an orgy, put it down. These things may not be realistic, but they will help lead you to something that is, something that represents who you really are, not who you were raised to be or were forced to be by circumstances.

It is okay to have more than three items but try for at least three. It is also okay to have items that are currently a part of your life, things that you would want to continue in your new paradigm.

Things I would like to do if could:

- _____
- _____
- _____
- _____
- _____
- _____
- _____
- _____
- _____
- _____
- _____
- _____

Looking Over the New Paradigm

If you've realized your life is great the way it is now, congratulations! That realization itself would be a worthwhile paradigm shift. Many of us are really quite content with what we have but succumb to other's beliefs about what we should strive for and make ourselves miserable trying to attain their wishes. A mother may feel pressured to have a career in addition to raising her family. A father may feel pressured to climb the corporate ladder rather than spending time with his family or favorite hobbies. Simply giving yourself permission to be yourself can be very difficult and very rewarding.

Probably though, you have at least something on your list that isn't a part of your life right now. Something that you deeply want, or believe that you want, and that will keep you from feeling good about yourself until you've at least given it a shot. The next step in this process is to think about whether or not your fat would be a barrier to that particular aspiration.

For each item, decide whether being fat is a barrier or not. Maybe you'd like to travel to distant places. Fat could definitely be a barrier; airplane seats are quite narrow and that would make fat a definite limitation. I've known people that are too fat even to see a movie in a theater because of the size of the seats.

In my case, I realized that I wanted to work as a consultant in the computer industry. It had been a dream since I'd gotten out of college but my experience with job interviews had taught me that being fat would almost immediately eliminate me from consideration. To most people it sent a message of lack of self-control and there was little I could do to correct that impression. So, for me, being fat was a definite barrier. Being interviewed was a big part of consulting and it was very unlikely that I could have much of a career as a consultant if nobody would hire me. To be a consultant at least some of the fat had to go.

Go back and *circle* any items on your list that would conflict with being fat. Again, if one of your items is something like "lose my fat" or "make more money", go back and define it further. Find a reason to lose your fat or a reason to make more money, something more specific. Get beyond the abstract ideas and think about things that would actually make you happy. Visualize yourself in this new life. Visualize how it would feel and how it would work. Ignore the present for now. The purpose of this exercise is to come up with your *own* reasons for losing fat and they must be specific, measurable reasons—something that you can someday ask yourself, "Is this what I am?"

Allowing for the Grief Cycle

So far, you have probably only developed vague ideas about what your current paradigm is and what you might like to change about it. However, I hope you have at least an idea of where you might like to head with your life. Remember that this is only a general direction. It will inevitably be modified as you move toward it.

Again I want to remind you of the grief cycle. Even when we want the paradigm to shift and welcome it, we must experience grief. Very likely, in the preceding exercise you've already felt some denial. Maybe you listed three components of a new paradigm but then quickly felt that they would be impossible. You might have felt that they would be fine for somebody else—someone with the talents or the finances or a different family situation—but not for you. Say hello to denial.

Perhaps you felt fear. We feel very vulnerable when a paradigm shifts or when we even contemplate making it shift. The very purpose of a paradigm is to allow us *not* to have to think about things; to filter out anything that is unimportant or threatening to us so that we are able to put our energy into other areas of our lives. We are supposed to take the paradigm for granted. When a paradigm is shown to be faulty, we are instantly exposed to a tremendous amount of information that we have no way to process.

It doesn't take a crisis to shift your paradigm. The only real shift is that you begin to believe in yourself and believe that you can have your life the way you want it. Be forewarned that when you attempt to change a paradigm yourself, it is all too easy to turn back when you experience any of the negative feelings associated with grief. In a crisis, there can be no turning back, so you are forced through the grief cycle. On your own however, you must fortify yourself to take steps forward, to stumble through that dark room towards the distant light coming from underneath the door, to allow yourself to be scared, stub your toes, get lost, but to keep moving anyway.

Recommendations

I would like to finish the section on paradigms with two recommended additional readings. The first is a fantastic novel, "She's Come Undone" by Wally Lamb. It is a gripping story following the life of a girl who suffers from an eating disorder. Written with a page-turning story line, it follows her from age four through adulthood. It is one of those books you can't put down once started. (Don't stop reading this one though!) Even though it is fiction, it truly does a fine job of showing how a person's life experiences and belief systems determine who they become. It allows the reader to observe paradigm shifts occurring in another person and allows a unique perspective about fat.

At one point in the story, an acquaintance recommends that Delores, the heroine, *acquire a taste for adventure.* That line has stuck in my mind since reading the book. It changes the perspective of shifting a paradigm. The key is to view the change as an adventure, a journey through unknown territory, to achieve a desired goal. I like to think of the movie "The Wizard of Oz" as a good analogy. Dorothy, the Scarecrow, Tin man, and Cowardly Lion all must fight their insecurities and weaknesses to find their way to their ultimate goal. For us, it makes tremendous entertainment, but to Dorothy, it is anything but fun! If you think about it, a lot of our entertainment uses this formula. It focuses on a hero fighting through unknown territory, overcoming fears and achieving a larger goal. Do you think part of the appeal of this type of story is that we desire to do the same thing for ourselves? Maybe we could all benefit by viewing ourselves as a character in a movie, struggling and scared, but never giving up.

The other recommendation I would like to make, is for you to seek out a recording by Canadian songwriter/singer, Jane Siberry. Her self-titled album titled *Jane Siberry* contains a song called "This Girl I Know". It captures the thought process of a fat person struggling with the fear of losing weight.

2

Agreements

Integrity

I once read about a cable TV company that was hooking up new customers to their system. A customer had called to make an appointment for an installation at 6:00 p.m., but the installer never showed up. The customer called back the next day and rescheduled another appointment for 6:00 p.m. Again, the same thing happened—no show. This happened several times when finally the irate customer pinned the customer service representative down—why was this happening? Why wasn't anybody showing up for the appointment? She replied, "Well, they only work until 5:00 p.m. I just make evening appointments because so many people want to schedule later times."

If you had a friend that had made a lunch date with you and then didn't keep it, how would you feel? Certainly if there were an emergency you'd understand, but what if it was merely that a better offer came along, something that was more appealing to your friend than you? Or, maybe your friend just didn't feel like meeting you that day. What would that say about your relationship and the value that your friend placed on it?

What if this happened repeatedly? How many times would you be willing to be stood up for a lunch date? How much evidence of your lack of importance in that person's life would you need before you abandoned the friendship?

Now, reverse the situation. What if you had a lunch date planned and something more appealing came up? Would you simply not show up for the lunch, leaving your friend sitting in the restaurant with no explanation? If it were truly an urgent conflict, you probably would contact your friend and ask for forgiveness. But, if it was something that just seemed like a better idea and you knew that your friend really was counting on meeting you, I suspect that you would honor the agreement with the friend and forgo the other offer. We recognize the value of a good friendship and are willing to make short-term sacrifices to maintain the long-term value.

Now think about what we do to ourselves. We want something, we make plans to get it, and then we quit. We stand ourselves up. It is as if we leave ourselves waiting in the restaurant with no explanation, the implication being that we have no importance or value to ourselves.

Maybe we need to get more physically fit. Maybe we need to lose some weight. Maybe we need to clean off our desks, get the oil changed in the car, update our resumes to begin a search for a better job, enroll in a night course, balance our checkbook, or simply floss our teeth. We all have an endless list of things we need to do. We all have plans to get those things done. However, all too frequently we never do them—or at least not until we are forced to.

We all have one friend who was with us when we were born, who will be with us when we die, and is with us for every moment in between: ourselves. There is one friend who will literally *always* be with us, and we treat this person with no respect. We make promises, we make plans, and then we stand ourselves up as we tacitly acknowledge that everything else in the world is more important. We let ourselves down with little or no explanation and it takes its toll. We become people we can't trust. We become people that say things that can't be believed. When it comes to ourselves we become liars. We become people that can't be counted on and we come to dislike ourselves, just as we would a friend that treated us the same way.

The customer service representative for the cable TV company in the example truly meant well. She had good intentions and wanted to keep her customers happy, but did she really do that in the end? Maybe the customers were happy when they were able to schedule an evening appointment, but were they happy when nothing was accomplished? What happened to their opinion of the company in the long run? How will they feel when they have to deal with the company in the future? Why bother to make plans that won't be kept?

Obviously, to lose weight, some degree of self-control is required. We make a plan to do something about it, maybe we even begin to implement the plan, and then we quit. This enforces the idea that we really are worthless or at least inferior to other people. Of course, we already knew that when we started. We never really expected to succeed; it was just another in a long line of good ideas.

For the fat person this is a double problem. Not only is the situation not corrected, but we also come to dislike ourselves—which usually makes us eat even more.

I always ended my diets with a colossal binge—an orgy of self-hate and self-punishment that was somehow strangely satisfying. It was as if I'd put the world back in order. I needed to undo anything that I'd accomplished and then usually do a little more damage just for good measure. I proved to myself once again just how worthless and weak I really was.

Will Power?

Of course, we all know why we do this to ourselves, why we can never accomplish what we know we should. We have no **WILL POWER!**

What is will power? It is thought of as strength of mind—the ability to carry out one's own wishes, desires, or plans. Seems like a reasonable definition but somewhat disturbing in that it sounds like an innate quality that you either have or you don't. And since I've never met anyone who believed that they had any, a better question might be *Where is Will Power?* Does anyone have it? Does it even exist?

Whatever it is, it seems that we are all tormented by our lack of it, and yet we seem willing to accept it as reason enough why we rarely accomplish what we want. We never wonder whether we can do anything to improve it. Why should we? It would be like trying to make yourself taller or shorter. We are what we are and we must live with that. Right?

So, as a substitute for will power, we turn to external sources of power to **force** us to do what we want. We look to diets to set rules for us, or friends and family to scold us when we stray from our plans. We spend a lot of money feeling that if we make that commitment it will somehow motivate us. We join health clubs or weight loss clinics to provide programs designed to isolate ourselves from temptation. We seek anything that comes from the *outside* to keep us "in line".

I met a woman in a group of fat people that I had spoken to who actually had tried having her jaws wired shut. She was extremely obese but quite attractive. She was intelligent with a fantastic wit and worked as a campaign manager for a local politician. She had everything going for her, but couldn't get rid of her fat. Eventually she found a doctor who was willing to perform the procedure. She told me of the fear she suffered before and after the operation. It had required a general anesthesia that made her nauseous after the procedure. She lived alone and had to spend a terrifying night worrying that she would vomit and suffocate because her jaw was wired shut. She had to carry a tool with her for emergency use to cut the wires if she started choking.

I thought that this was the most amazing story; a person who wanted to be thin so badly that she was willing to endure pure hell and risk her life to obtain it. But, even if the wires had worked (they didn't, she cut them out) what could be expected later? Was she going to go through life with her jaw wired shut? If she got thin, would she then have the self-control to maintain the thinness? If she had to rely on a physical barrier to enforce her wishes, how could she realistically expect to maintain her goal? What *was* her goal?

I wish I could report that she learned the techniques presented here and that her life has been fantastic ever since. The truth is she never came back to the class after the first session. I think I saw in her eyes a glimmer of understanding but also such tremendous self-doubt and self-loathing that the idea of facing those issues was more horrifying than the night with the wire cutters had been.

I know of people who make bets or otherwise spend tremendous amounts of money on diet programs simply to "up the ante" so that somehow they will find the motivation to succeed. But no source of surrogate will power has ever been discovered. If our own wants and desires aren't enough motivation, why bother? What can possibly be more important to us than that? In reality, *everything but* our own wants and desires seem to be more important to us, or so we think. And *that* is the real problem.

Will power is the ability to carry out one's own wishes and desires, not someone else's. However, I believe that whenever there is a lack of will power, without realizing it, we have substituted other people's wishes for our own.

Because we are social creatures, we tend to value and genuinely need the acceptance of others. Their opinions are important, but so are our own. And history is full of examples of widely loved people who are never truly happy with themselves.

I believe that we must first know and love ourselves before we can seek the love of others. We may actually find someone who loves us just as we are, but we can never feel truly happy if this love is completely external to us and does not reflect how we feel about ourselves.

Total self-love without the love and approval of others would not be satisfying either. A balance is required. The problem comes because of the reality that other people's desires (with respect to us) tend to be more defined than our own. Because of this, we readily adopt their ideas as our own. We have little practice determining what *we really want* for ourselves.

But these "wants" do exist for each of us, whether or not we are conscious of them, and if they are at cross-purposes with our external environment and stated plans we will unconsciously sabotage ourselves.

The main problem with the definition of will power is that it is defined as a noun, a thing. It isn't. It is a verb, a behavior, an action. It isn't something we have, it is something we do. And we all do it perfectly; we just don't know our own wills.

Agreements—A Power Tool

There is an old saying, "When all you have is a hammer, the whole world looks like a nail." We can only approach life with the tools that we have in our tool kit, so we can only deal with problems in ways that we have already tried. If the job really calls for a wrench and all we have is a hammer, the temptation is to use the hammer in place of the wrench—with predictably lousy results.

Now, think of all that you know about managing your weight as a hammer and what the job really calls for is a wrench. You can bash away with tremendous force, cursing and struggling with your task, but the results are going to be limited at best. You need a wrench.

If you learn nothing else from this book, focus on the concept of *agreements*. I consider the agreement technique by far the most useful tool in the entire methodology and an important addition to your tool kit for handling life. Agreements are useful in all areas of your life, not merely in dealing with fat. For example, I have used agreements to learn to play the piano, study a foreign language, clean off a messy desk, and to fill out my tax return. Anytime I find myself lacking "will power", I know that I need to use an agreement.

Agreements are what you will use to re-establish your damaged relationship with yourself, and in the process, take on much larger tasks that genuinely mean something to you.

The technique is deceptively simple. You say to yourself: "I agree to _____ by _____", filling in the blanks with the "what" and the "when" of your specific task. This phrase becomes a trigger to your unconscious mind that you are committed to this particular undertaking and will allow *nothing* to prevent you from completing it. And I mean *absolutely nothing!*

You must learn to make only agreements that you truly intend to keep. You will learn to recognize them as deadly serious and nothing to be taken lightly. You will realize that this is *you* counting on *you*, and *to let yourself down will cause damage that will be extremely difficult to repair.*

Picture a young, innocent, and trusting child, maybe a little 5-year-old girl that you have agreed to pick up after school. You've told her to be waiting at the street and that you will be by to pick her up at 3:30. Now, a more appealing offer comes along at 3:15, something you'd much rather do than pick her up, say a chance to meet some friends. What do you do? Would you really leave the child standing on the street with no explanation? Think of the effect that would have on her. She would be nervous at first, then scared, then terrified as she stood waiting and waiting, hoping that you would keep your promise as the darkness of the evening approached. Maybe you truly enjoyed the time with your friends, but would it be worth it when you consider the trauma that you've inflicted on this little child?

Or maybe something nobler than an offer from a friend comes along. Let's say your boss asks you to work late and take on something critical to your job, something that is very important to the company as well as your career. What do you do then? Do you leave the child standing on the street? Do you get a message to her that something really important came up and you can't pick her up today, but you promise to be there tomorrow? What good would that do? I'm sure she'll take comfort in that as the darkness surrounds her. Of course you don't do that, you work it out. You tell your boss that you have an urgent situation that you can't avoid. Maybe you pick her up and then return to work to finish the assignment. Maybe you take the work home and work late into the night if necessary. But you certainly don't abandon a small child.

What if you know that the traffic will be bad at that time of day and that making the pick-up on time might be difficult? Do you show up late? Hopefully in making your agreement you've taken that into consideration and you will leave early enough to keep the agreed upon appointment.

Certainly, even with the best intentions, things can go wrong. You might turn down the friend's offer, explain the situation to your boss, leave work early enough to beat the traffic, and then be in an automobile accident. But, I suspect that even then, as they were lifting you on a stretcher into the ambulance, you'd find a way to communicate your problem to the paramedic and arrange for some alternative solution for the child waiting on the street corner.

When making agreements with yourself, you need to picture that innocent little child. No excuses will be good enough to explain away the trauma that you'd inflict if you broke the agreement. This is serious business. Picture yourself as a child, young and innocent. Think of the way you were long before the world had a chance to toughen you and teach you to expect disappointment. Think of *yourself* when you were naive and trusting. That is the person that you will be making agreements with. That is who you will be hurting if you don't keep your word. That is who will be injured if left standing alone in the darkness.

Finding Your Current Level of Trustworthiness

Probably your current level of *personal* trustworthiness is quite low. Perhaps you make agreements with yourself and ignore them within minutes. More than likely, you are very good about keeping agreements with others, but when you need to do something for yourself, forget it. If anything, you've trained yourself to agree to what you know you *won't* do, not the opposite.

This is the root of a tremendous amount of self-contempt, even though we are rarely conscious of it. That little child inside of us has become abused and probably finds ways to fight back and make our lives miserable. Since you are reading this book, chances are you abuse food in some way. You are probably wondering why you can't control yourself, why you eat when you're not hungry, why you eat to the point of physical pain.

Eating is very pleasant, but most food abusers go way beyond pleasure. I can remember eating so much that all I could do was lie on the couch with my pants unbuttoned after a binge. A binge might have started out pleasantly, but it certainly ended up in pain. Could it be that the little child inside of me was angry about being abandoned? Maybe he'd found a way to get back at me.

It is important to realize your current state of mental fitness. Don't think of it as an illness. Don't classify yourself as somebody who is different or deficient. Think of your brain as a muscle that is out of shape but quite capable of getting stronger.

Let's pretend you wanted to try bodybuilding. Picture yourself going into a gym where a selection of barbells for weight lifting is available. They range from tiny ones weighing less than a pound up to some that weigh 200 pounds. Which one would you grab hold of first: one of the big ones, or the tiny ones? Chances are you'd grab hold of one of the smaller ones and try it tentatively, being careful not to injure yourself. If it were too heavy, you'd put it back and try a lighter one. If it were too light, you'd switch to a larger one.

Through trial and error, you'd find your current level of strength and begin building from that point. I doubt that you would look around the gym to see what other people were lifting to determine where you should start. If somebody was lifting 100 pounds, that should mean absolutely nothing to you as far as your level of fitness goes. It is totally unrelated. *You are where you are. Anybody else's level of fitness is meaningless.*

Attempting a diet is the equivalent of running into the gym and grabbing hold of the 200-pound barbell. You might be able somehow drag it off the rack, but you would have limited success with it. If you were lucky, you'd probably only drop it on your toe. If you were less lucky, you might injure your back and wind up in worse shape than when you started. The last thing you should do is lower your opinion of yourself, simply because you couldn't lift a 200-pound barbell.

Agreements are like mental barbells. You start where you are and you build up to stronger levels. You don't worry about where you are with respect to other people. The *only* place you can begin is where *you* are.

Use the barbells as metaphor for agreements. Start small and build up. Let the muscles develop. Fairly quickly, you will find your agreement fitness improving. For most people, keeping their word with themselves is a new and invigorating experience. They find out quickly that they are just as good as anyone and quickly begin to move on to higher levels of mental fitness, passing others along the way.

Start by choosing an extremely simple agreement. It can even be trivial and pointless. For example, say to yourself, "I agree to stand up and count to 10, right now" and then do it. Try it now. Say it first and then follow through.

Did you try it? If you did, great! However, I'll bet that many people reading this won't be able to do it. They may make excuses like "I know that I could do it, so I don't need to" or "I would feel silly" or "I don't see the point, all I'm looking for is someone to tell me what to eat". In their minds, they think they are accomplishing something, but in reality, they are damaging themselves. Something as simple as making and acting upon that agreement may be way beyond their level of fitness.

If you tried the agreement and succeeded, you probably need to move to a heavier barbell. But if you didn't, then think of something easier that you can agree to and feel successful with. The main point is to *set yourself up for success* and begin to establish credibility again with that little child.

Don't take on what you know is too much. When you say the words "I agree to _____ by _____", you must know that you mean it and can count on yourself to do it absolutely, with no exceptions. The little child is waiting for you. It won't work to let her down today but promise to be there tomorrow. And it certainly doesn't make any sense to say "I agree to pick you up", but not say *when*. That doesn't do anybody any good. All agreements must be time specific or you will find yourself quickly making excuses and ignoring the whole process.

This simple technique will become the core of your new life. You will become a person with integrity and it will spread to all areas of your life. You will feel a new affection for yourself, and as you get stronger, much of the self-abuse will begin to lessen.

Try It Three Times a Day

I can't prescribe exactly how you should begin using agreements simply because I can't predict your current level of fitness. However, as a starting point I suggest you make three simple agreements a day and see how you do with them. In other words, I'd like you to make an agreement with yourself now to make three additional agreements in a 24-hour period. These should be three things that you know you could do using your level of fitness right now. They probably should be trivial and certainly shouldn't be very difficult (no more than the equivalent of 1-pound barbells). In the beginning, it is very, very important to be totally successful with your agreements. You are training yourself just as you might teach a pet a new trick or a child how to do a new task. You must find a logical approach based on only your own level of ability. That theme will occur throughout this book.

Everything you learn needs to be tempered with your own particular reality and situation. The skill that you are developing is to be able to assess your current situation and create a solution for that moment in time—all the time keeping your ultimate goal in mind. Know what you want, lay out a plan to get there, and then execute the plan.

To begin with, just work on training yourself to respond to the words "I agree to _____ by _____", just as you would expect a pet dog to respond to the command, "sit".

Agreements need to be to "*do*" something, never to "*not do*" something. We can train ourselves to make something happen, but it is difficult to stop something without displacing it with something else. If you want to agree to prevent something, engineer an agreement that displaces or delays the behavior rather than just avoiding it.

Animal trainers know that it is very difficult (if not impossible) to train an animal to stop doing something. Instead, they teach an alternative to the activity (such as teaching a dog chew on an appropriate toy rather than try to teach it *not* to chew on the furniture). We certainly are more complex beings than animals, but not all that much more complex if you really think about it. Our nature is to learn to do new things and not to stop doing things we already know how to do.

Agreements need to be short term, especially in the beginning. You can't realistically agree to things too far into the future because many things can change your plans. Start by agreeing to something in the next few minutes. If you are successful, try agreeing to something in the next hour. As you get better, try making an agreement in the morning for something in the afternoon. This will probably be somewhat more difficult. What seemed simple in the morning can easily become insurmountable later in the day due to the effects of stress, exhaustion, and unforeseen obligations.

Time has a way of eroding agreements, so be careful but firm. The longer the period of time, the more vulnerable the agreement is to failure. As you get stronger, you will be able to cast agreements out further into the future. But start small.

Experiment to find your level of strength. Notice when you fail. Is it the time of day? Is the length of time between making the agreement and carrying it out? Is it the subject matter of the agreement? Is it when you are tired or hungry?

I strongly urge you to stay away from food agreements in the beginning of this process. For most of us, that is such an emotional area that even what would appear to be simple agreements are all but impossible. I remember originally trying to agree that I would leave one bite of food on my plate uneaten. I could eat whatever and as much as I wanted, but I had to leave one bite. I could take as large of a helping as I needed to be "full", but I had to leave one extra bite on my plate. However, even with such a "loose" agreement, I couldn't keep it. My mind just wouldn't let me leave something on my plate that I wanted to eat.

How to Break Your Agreements

There seems to be no end to the ways our minds have to break their agreements. The creativity is unbounded, but most techniques fall into some basic categories:

- Forgetting
- Trivialization
- Vanity
- Diminished Importance
- Partial performance
- Postponement
- Priority Conflict
- Lack of Energy

Let's start with a trivial agreement and think of all the ways it might be broken. For example, let's say that you agree to stand up and count to ten out loud exactly one hour from now, but an hour from now you forget. A lot of us will use "forgetting" as a way to sabotage the agreement.

You may need to design your agreements so that you can't forget. You might have to invest in a cheap $5 watch with a timer that can be set to beep when it is time for you to keep your agreement. A truly stubborn "forgetter" will "forget" to go to the store to buy one. If the forgetter already has a watch with a timer, they might tend to "forget" to set it, or wear it.

Or, maybe you decide that the $5 investment in the watch is not worth it, or that counting to ten cannot possibly be of any value. You later might find yourself using the excuse that you need to make more meaningful agreements (trivialization) and will try that instead.

Or, if somebody came into the room just when it was time to count, you might feel too embarrassed to do such a thing in front of someone else so you break the agreement (vanity).

Maybe somebody with a conflicting request for your time comes along and you feel this person has needs that supersede your own. Certainly, someone else's requirements for your time must always be of a higher value than your own (diminished importance).

Another great agreement breaking technique is to only do part of the agreement, maybe count to ten but not bother to stand up when doing it, or skip some of the numbers, or not say them out loud (partial performance).

Perhaps, when the chosen time arrives, you decide that an another hour later might actually be a *better* time to "keep" the agreement (postponement) so you renew rather than keep the agreement—just like renewing a library book that you keep intending to read but never quite get around to.

Some of us unconsciously make conflicting agreements. Just when it's time to count to ten, it "turns out" that it is also time make a phone call that you also agreed to make (priority conflict).

Maybe you were just plain "too tired" to keep the agreement. It seemed like a reasonable agreement when you made it, but you didn't know how exhausted you were going to feel when the actual time to keep the agreement came (lack of energy).

You probably can invent an entirely new category of agreement breaking techniques. Nevertheless, whenever you fail, pay attention to how you break your agreements. This is when you meet the enemy. This is when that nasty demon inside you with such contempt will make itself visible.

Your job is to flush the demon out into the open and learn all you can about him. You want to do battle on your own terms with your own rules. That is why it is so important for you to create your *own* agreements rather than accepting my suggestions or anyone else's. This is also is why you should stay away from food agreements in the beginning. This test needs to be conducted in a controlled environment and food is usually too emotionally loaded to evaluate the agreement process objectively.

You are developing a skill. You are in boot camp and you aren't ready to go into battle with the demon just yet. Your goal now is simply to learn about him and build yourself up to deal with him when the battles come later on.

Respect other people in your life, but be very clear that they cannot be your number one priority. When you have made an agreement—that is all there is to it. There is *nothing more to be said* about it. It is a commitment with a higher purpose. You either keep it or you don't. It isn't something you *can't have opinions* about. You must be clear on your performance. Did you keep the agreement? That is always a "yes or no" question; no explanations can undo the damage of a broken agreement. To break the agreement is to systematically injure yourself and to leave that little child waiting in the dark. Never lose sight of that.

"Kept" Agreements Are Energizing

There is a strange thing that happens when you keep an agreement, particularly one that you weren't sure you *could* keep. Frequently you will be hit with a sudden burst of energy. Rather than being tired, you get a jolt of energy when the weight has been lifted that you've been carrying—a weight that you may not have been aware of. This is the weight of procrastination, self-doubt, and denial. You begin to realize that you are a very good person and actually start building a healthier relationship with yourself. As you get better, you will coincidentally stop abusing yourself, at least as much or as often. You start to become somebody that you can trust.

If you have ever played the video game "Pac Man", think of the little power pills that the Pac Man could eat. Once he ate one, all of the ghosts that were chasing him now ran in fear and he could in turn devour them instead. An agreement is very much like one of those little power pills. It isn't always easy to get to, but once you "consume" it you are granted a lot of energy to take on the world.

The energy will only last for a while and then you must continue to seek new sources as your strength increases. Your level of trustworthiness will increase until you stop exercising it, and then it will begin to decrease. This is not something that you can do for a short period of time and then quit.

But don't think about "forever", just think about the next few hours. At this point, the thought of keeping agreements for the rest of your life probably feels overwhelming. However, what you haven't experienced yet is the shot of energy that you will get along the way when you keep a challenging agreement. This will change your outlook completely. You will get to know your new self and see yourself in an entirely new way—and in a new paradigm. Don't let the past ruin the future.

Where to Use Your New Tool

I have come to use agreements in every aspect of my life. I've used them to teach myself to play the piano, learn a foreign language, and finish writing this book. Anytime I feel the desire to accomplish something but just can't keep moving with my task, I use agreements. They are a fantastic tool to remove any obstacles in my path.

I've learned that when I use those magic words "I agree…" whatever other self-defeating ideas I have simply no longer apply. I respond to the agreement without question, overriding my conscious or unconscious protests.

I do suggest that you initially develop this technique in areas of your life that aren't related to eating—at least not with what and how much you eat, as in the form of a diet. Later on as you get stronger, you might try to modify your eating behavior slightly.

One of my early agreements was not to eat anything when I got home from work until after I'd changed clothes. My usual behavior was to walk in the door, and before I'd even set my briefcase down, I'd yank open the door of the refrigerator and start eating. Rather than agree to *not* do that (remember that agreements to *not* do something are all but impossible to keep), I agreed to wait just a little bit until I was in more comfortable clothes. Then I was free to do whatever I wanted. Somehow, that extra 10 minutes coupled with my feeling of taking control of the situation made my assault on the refrigerator just a little bit more manageable and gave me the strength to avoid an all out binge.

When you are facing a defeating form of behavior, it is better to replace it or deflect it slightly than to try to agree not to do it. We really can't think in terms of negatives, only positives. Agree to get out of bed 10 minutes earlier for example, rather than agree *not* be late for work.

I would also recommend that you avoid agreements that require the participation of other people. As much as possible, you want to have complete control over the outcome and mixing another person's will into your agreements tends to cause problems.

For example, you might agree to take a walk tomorrow morning, but don't make the agreement specifically include your best friend. That doesn't mean when the time comes that your friend can't come along, you just don't want your feelings to be influenced by someone else. If your friend decides that driving over to the Dunkin' Donuts seems like a better idea than walking, you don't want to see your agreement crumbling before your eyes. You simply say that you are going for a walk and that they are welcome to come along. After you are done, maybe you will be interested in Dunkin' Donuts, but the agreement comes first.

Initially, your agreements are probably best if they are not associated with any particular goal. You're really just learning the technique. It is best to choose areas that are not sensitive for you. Don't start with tasks that you've been putting off for years. Easy and unusual agreements seem to work best. Agree to wear your watch on the other wrist. Agree to wear your glasses instead of your contact lenses. Agree to wear your underwear inside out. It doesn't matter, just as long as you can objectively decide whether you kept the agreement or not. Entertain yourself with nonsense agreements. The overall goal at first is simply to train yourself to respond.

When you are comfortable with the agreement concept, start trying things in areas that are associated with a particular goal. For example, in learning to play the piano, I would agree just to sit at the keyboard for 10 minutes. It wasn't necessary to play. The next day I might agree to play just one particular measure in a piece of music 10 times. After I accomplished my agreement, I was free to stop. I didn't worry about whether or not I was making progress fast enough. I made an agreement. I kept it. Period.

Oddly, in most cases I wouldn't just get up and leave the piano after I'd kept the agreement. I would typically feel filled with a rush of energy and spend more time practicing. Once I'd smashed through a simple barrier I was back in control and full of ideas.

Don't be discouraged if you keep your agreements but have no further desire to lose weight. At some point, you may want to examine your true intentions and decide whether they are truly yours or someone else's, but save that until you have genuinely tried and succeeded repeatedly with small agreements.

In my case, playing the piano was something that I'd always wanted to be able to do. Once I started feeling in control, I was eager to continue with the process. However, if my only real desire to play had come from a parent who "planted" that seed years before when I was child, I doubt that any quantity of agreements would have gotten me much closer to my goal.

Intentions, Goals, and Tasks

Accomplishing anything provides some degree of pleasure. Getting my taxes finished by April 15 certainly fills me with a sense of relief, but it is hardly something I would do if I had the choice.

Agreements are useful in all areas of life, both with the goals that we personally have and the goals that we are given (for example the ones given by the IRS). Sometimes agreements are useful simply to remove roadblocks that will ultimately free us to work on what we truly want. Even along the path to a goal that we want, we may have to agree to things we'd rather not be doing. If the path were an easy one we'd already be there.

However, really to feel good in life we must have goals that we want for ourselves. To do this we must be clear about our *intentions*. I think of an intention as a general direction we'd like to head. Within that direction, there are probably multiple *goals* that relate to the intention. To attain a goal, there are probably multiple *tasks* to be performed. Agreements are used to accomplish these tasks.

The larger picture is that agreements are used to accomplish tasks, which are used to accomplish goals, which fulfill our intentions.

Agreements >>> Tasks >>> Goals >>> Intentions

Most fat people have the goal of losing weight, but they are rarely clear on their intentions. Somehow being fat comes with the notion that we shouldn't be. It is a part of our culture and we accept it as a given. However, chances are that the very root of our fat is that we want something completely different from what we have. Becoming thin in our current lives isn't likely to change anything.

I have talked with hundreds of fat people and rarely can they explain what it is that they really want out of being thin. Somehow, they want to change *everything*, but accomplish this by changing *nothing*. Fear typically holds them in place when coupled with a paradigm that tells them that it probably isn't possible anyway.

I didn't start losing weight until I realized that what I wanted was respect in my profession. I knew I was good—very good actually—and I knew that nobody was going to take me seriously if I was fat. Fat people have no self-control, how can they be good at anything? I thought this couldn't be true, but at some level, I wasn't so sure. Not only was I fat, but I had a life filled with other unaccomplished tasks. Maybe my perception of me wasn't all that faulty. Maybe I really had no self-control in any area of my life.

Instead of "losing" something, I started thinking in terms of "gaining" something—self-respect. I started creating the person that I wanted to be. I became clear about my intentions, I set goals within those intentions, I saw the tasks necessary to achieve the goals, and I made agreements to get there.

The whole notion of *losing weight* is ridiculous; we need to think in terms of what we are *gaining!*

Life is a journey. It may help to think of intentions as a road trip with goals as the cities along the way, tasks as the roads you choose to get to the cities, and agreements as the vehicle you are traveling in.

It is perfectly okay to change your intentions. Mine have changed frequently over the years particularly as I learn to separate my own intentions from the ones imposed by other people. Later you may find that the goals that you have set within an intention are not the best route. You may find that it might be more interesting to route your journey through a completely different city. Moreover, it is okay to choose different tasks to get to a particular goal. Sometimes the roads that you've chosen turn out not to be the best, or you might learn of new routes along the way that are more suited to your journey.

And never forget the vehicle you are traveling in—the agreement. It will need constant attention. If you get out of the habit of making agreements you will need to build yourself back up. If you notice yourself slipping a little too much, it is time for an agreement tune-up. As agreement fitness diminishes, other people's intentions tend to creep in making things even more confusing.

Other People in Our Lives

Other people that are a part of our lives are certainly a priority for most of us. Our intentions probably include having a good family life and friends. There is no reason that goals can't be set that allow for and include these people. However, be forewarned that as supportive as people might seem, as you become stronger they will inevitably feel threatened and might even work unconsciously to thwart your efforts.

In addition, I've noticed that my tolerance for people who don't keep their word has dropped considerably. I was surrounded by friends that supported the "old" me and they really weren't too thrilled with the "new" one. The things that we had in common started to vanish and the relationships suffered.

In time, I made new friends that were more suited to my new life. But that in itself is a little frightening. The temptation to abandon my intentions and return to the old ways was strong at times. The new friends were living lives that were foreign to me, and the old friends had developed resentment. There were times that I felt quite isolated. I had to focus on was my intentions and where my ultimate destination was.

Family members are another story. They are even more affected by changes in our lives. We are a part of their lives, and they might not be so eager to have their life changed.

My marriage of 14 years ended. My wife wasn't married to the same person anymore. The new person that I became probably wouldn't have been of much interest to her had our first meeting come for the first time after my transformation.

Don't just assume that if you get more physically attractive that your relationship will improve. However, I'm certainly not suggesting that it won't. There is certainly no reason to think that a relationship shouldn't find new life if one of the participants finds a new life and becomes happier with life in general. Nevertheless, I can almost guarantee that it will be affected in some way. Be prepared!

Disaster Recovery

A big component of the agreement process is to forgive yourself when appropriate. I know of nobody who has a 100% success rate with agreements. In fact, if someone did, I would be quite sure that they weren't really striving to improve themselves. If you're not failing occasionally, you aren't trying hard enough. At the same time, this reality isn't meant to be a valid excuse to get out of the agreement. There are **NO EXCUSES**. Always remember either an agreement is kept or it isn't. Nothing changes that.

The trick in developing a good agreement technique is to know how to deal with the results of an agreement. You must look into yourself and decide what your level of fitness is and how you want to respond to the outcome of the agreement. If you succeed, do you need to increase the difficulty, or are you happy with your current level of fitness? If you fail, do you need to lower the difficulty or just fine tune the original agreement so that you can succeed?

Life is a dynamic environment; it never works to approach with a static set of rules, particularly somebody else's rules. In a sense, a diet is a static set of agreements that you are handed to adopt into your life. This makes the chances for success almost nonexistent since it has nothing to do with your life and your circumstances.

When I used to diet, I fell victim to the "week" concept. In one particular diet that I favored, I would start out each week with my meal plan and great intentions. There were a few things on the diet that I actually liked, but I was also supposed to eat something like five broiled "fish meals" and one "liver meal" each week. Now, guess which things I ate first in the week. The liver? Hardly. I started by using up all of the things I liked. By Wednesday, all I had left was liver and broiled fish. Guess what happened! I'd decide to wait until next Monday to *really* get serious about this diet. I knew that this was going to be a tough week anyway and the last thing I wanted to be doing was eating liver when I had all of this stress in my life. So, I would just decide to give up on the rest of the week and start over. I had no plan to deal with failure even though it happened every week.

The key concept is this: **There is no starting over!** There is no week to begin, no Monday to start with, no period of time to wait to try again. When you slip, you are still in the game. Right then, right now. *Failing is part of suc-*

ceeding. The only rules are the ones that you make. You must be clear about your overall intentions, i.e. your new paradigm and where you are in your journey to get there. When your car runs off the road, do whatever it takes to get it back on the road. Immediately!

I had an image in my mind that if I went off the diet, it was over until next Monday. I believed that if I lost control and had a binge, somehow that should put an end to things. It was over. My car had a flat tire. My journey was over until I could begin again, which meant hitching a ride back to the start and getting a new car. It never crossed my mind to simply change the tire and use the spare.

All of this self-defeating behavior was quite predictable, of course. In the first place, the diet never had anything to do with *my life* or how *I lived*. It didn't come from me, it came from somebody else's ideas about how I should behave. It was a package of agreements that I didn't create but accepted nevertheless.

When you make an agreement, make sure you have some idea of what you will do if you fail. This doesn't mean plan to fail, just don't fail to plan. Be prepared to forgive yourself if you make a mistake, and then develop a new approach that deals with the problem. You can't foresee every possible thing that could go wrong, but you can accept the notion that when things do go wrong you will still keep going. Having a flat tire doesn't terminate the journey—you solve the problem and keep heading towards your destination. No matter what the disaster, you plan to recover and continue the journey.

Agreement Exercise

Try to think of three agreements for the next 24-hour period. This may be too difficult at this point and you might have to settle for only one or two, but try for three. They can be anything that you might not normally do—something that you wouldn't automatically do in your daily routine. They can be trivial and pointless, or something useful that you've been putting off (but beware of the 200-pound barbell; this isn't the time to decide to clean out the garage that you've been ignoring for years!).

Choose something that you feel you have a reasonable chance to keep. Don't set yourself up for failure, but be prepared to deal with it if it comes. Write the agreements down. Put down the specifics. At the end of the 24-hour period check off whether you kept the agreement or not. Check "yes" or "no". Remember there can be no other answer. If you failed, try to identify the category of excuse that you used. Look for a pattern of failure. If you did keep the agreement, pat yourself on the back!

After completing one day of agreements, make agreements for the next day based on the results of the previous. If your agreements were too hard, make easier ones. If they were too easy, make harder ones. If you recognize a pattern in your agreement breaking, design your agreements to address that problem. But, always be honest with yourself! This isn't a time to play games. You can genuinely injure your self-esteem if you don't play fair with yourself. Don't abandon that little child on the street corner.

I've included a section to write down agreements for several days, but always focus only on the coming day. Use a different sheet of paper if you need more room, but you must write your agreement down specifically so that you can evaluate it afterwards.

It is okay to repeat the same agreements on subsequent days, but make sure you're not kidding yourself by choosing overly easy agreements. Keep the picture of the barbells in mind. Be realistic about where you are and when you need to move to a higher level.

I've also included a list of suggestions to use in formulating your agreements. They are not suggestions of actual agreements because those must come from you and your personal life, but they should give you some guidelines in setting up your agreements. In addition, there is a list of common excuses used to get out of agreements. It may help you cope with the demon who inevitably will try to thwart your efforts. If you consider how you might be inclined to break an agreement in advance, you can be prepared to avoid disaster. Think about which ones are you most likely to use.

Don't make agreements for more than one 24-hour period. Don't agree to things several days in advance. You will develop the ability to make longer agreements as you get stronger, but be careful in the beginning and focus on the short term. Set yourself up for success. Adopt this process into your everyday life. Keep making agreements and increasing their difficulty until you are happy with your level of fitness. Soon you should find yourself able to take on even the most nagging tasks simply by agreeing to do them. Once you have made this commitment it will cease to be an object for debate, the case will be closed. You've agreed; you perform. You will find that the job is rarely as difficult as all of the energy you put into avoiding it. In fact, after you complete it, invariably you will be hit with a burst of energy once you are free of all of the internal debate, denial, and procrastination.

Don't stop this process when you've filled up the following pages. The agreement concept will be incorporated into the complete Cornerstone methodology and you will have many opportunities to use the tool in each subject area as well in other places in your life. Keep working on agreements and developing your ability as you continue reading about the Four Cornerstones.

Date: _____

Agreement	To be completed when?	Kept? (Yes/No)	Excuse (if broken)

Date: _____

Agreement	To be completed when?	Kept? (Yes/No)	Excuse (if broken)

Date: _____

Agreement	To be completed when?	Kept? (Yes/No)	Excuse (if broken)

Date: _____

Agreement	To be completed when?	Kept? (Yes/No)	Excuse (if broken)

Date: _____

Agreement	To be completed when?	Kept? (Yes/No)	Excuse (if broken)

Date: _____

Agreement	To be completed when?	Kept? (Yes/No)	Excuse (if broken)

Date: _____

Agreement	To be completed when?	Kept? (Yes/No)	Excuse (if broken)

Date: _____

Agreement	To be completed when?	Kept? (Yes/No)	Excuse (if broken)

Date: _____

Agreement	To be completed when?	Kept? (Yes/No)	Excuse (if broken)

Suggestions

- Use the phrase "I agree to ____ by ____" as key words to yourself that you are extremely serious about this.

- Avoid agreements concerning food, at least initially.

- Be clear about your intentions. Keep your destination in mind.

- Start with trivial agreements then proceed to harder ones.

- Think of the little child that is counting on you to keep your agreement.

- Visualize your brain as a muscle getting stronger.

- Strive for an 80%–90% success rate; don't get caught in a perfectionism/procrastination loop.

- Break larger goals into manageable agreements.

- Visualize yourself keeping the agreement.

- Externalize agreements by writing them or confiding in someone.

- Have a "disaster recovery" plan.

- Visualize yourself recovering if the worst happens.

- Acquire a taste for adventure!

Favorite Excuses

- I have no willpower.

- I forgot.

- Something more important came up and I didn't have the time.

- I had to modify the agreement to fit the circumstances.

- I could only keep part of the agreement.

- I'll trying making agreements later when my life is less hectic.

- I haven't broken my agreement; I just haven't kept it yet.

Add your favorite excuses here!

- _____
- _____
- _____
- _____
- _____
- _____
- _____
- _____
- _____
- _____
- _____
- _____

3

The Cornerstone Concept

The Cornerstone Infrastructure

Ironically, at some point during my fat years I had experimented with each of the four Cornerstones in one way or another. Each of them stands on its own merit, and each is advocated by its own group of supporters. Interestingly, none of them is usually thought of as having much to do with weight loss with the possible exception of the Fitness Cornerstone.

I had heard of them all, usually in conjunction with a diet, and saw their individual value but I was never able to make them a permanent part of my life. I would do my best to adopt the various techniques, but I inevitably would lose interest and drop the habit. It wasn't until I took Dr. Bradley's course and learned to think of these concepts supporting each other rather than standing alone that everything clicked into place.

Each of the Cornerstones affects a specific area of your life, but also interacts with the others to form an infrastructure to improve the quality of your life. As your interest in one particular Cornerstone might begin to wane, the others will give you the support necessary to continue working towards your ultimate goal.

One Cornerstone might seem harder than the others, but which one is the hardest will vary from person to person. In addition, at different times each of the Cornerstones might seem more difficult simply because the particular area of life that the Cornerstone addresses might be causing problems. This is when the other three will provide the support necessary to deal with the situation rather than give up.

Meet the Cornerstones

The four Cornerstones are:

- Journal Keeping

- Stress Reduction

- Fitness

- Nutrition

Each of them will be discussed in detail in the following sections. At this point the important thing is to realize that each of the Cornerstones is *equally* important. Each provides its own value while supporting the others.

Think of them as the four sides of a building. They combine to provide a solid enclosure for living *your* life the way *you* want. They will ultimately become routine habits that will help you through the roughest moments in life, and they will give you the tool necessary to achieve whatever you decide that you want for yourself.

In a sense, the agreement technique that we have just learned will provide the mortar to cement the Cornerstones together. Agreements will be used within each of the four Cornerstones to develop that particular area.

You will inevitably be better at some of the Cornerstones than at others. This is normal. What is hard for one person might seem easy for another. Don't compare yourself to anybody else. Use your successes in one Cornerstone to encourage successes in the others. Pay particular attention to the areas that are difficult. This is valuable information. It will serve to highlight what is going on in your life that is the root of your frustrations. The temptation will be to focus all of your energy on your easier Cornerstones. Don't be seduced by this. You need support from all four areas to make the progress that you truly desire.

I have also seen people do an adequate job in each of the four areas, but make no real progress overall. These are people that have not clearly defined their intentions and haven't been able to look past their old paradigm. If you don't have a general sense about what it is you want to change in your life, there isn't much chance that you will be able to change anything. Even if that is the case, you will feel better by using the Cornerstones to improve your general quality of life as it is today.

Certainly, there is value in implementing the Cornerstones even if you are already perfectly happy with your life. Anyone will experience an increase in the overall sense of well-being by adding the Cornerstone infrastructure as a daily routine. But those who choose to erect their Cornerstones in a new paradigm will see quantum improvements and experience a complete redefinition of who they are.

Forget about losing weight. Think about replacing it. Think about the new person you identified when you learned about paradigms. Realize that the only limitations are the ones imposed by your current paradigm. If you decide to live in a new paradigm, there doesn't need to be any limitations.

People frequently ask me how long it took me to lose all of my weight. When I was first asked that question, it caught me by surprise. I actually had no idea how long it had taken. When I thought about it, it seemed as if it had happened in an instant. I heard about the Cornerstones, realized that this was what I was seeking, and that was all there was to it. I became clear about who I wanted to become, and from that moment forward, I started living the life of that new person. It seemed that in less than a minute I became somebody else. Of course I still had the fat, but it began disappearing—it just didn't have anything to do with the new me. I never had a goal weight. I never chose some point in the distance that would indicate that life could begin. I simply started living the new life.

What I could accomplish within each of the Cornerstones was limited at first, but it really didn't matter. I knew that I would improve in each of the areas, and that even a slight improvement was all that was important. Besides, I was becoming who I wanted to be and everything else would fall in line with that. I didn't think of myself as somebody who was on the outside looking in, I was simply on the inside growing within the new context of my life. I liked myself much more and began to trust myself. I gave up worrying about someone else's goals for me and began choosing my own.

Be Prepared for Change

Obviously, you are not going to be able to have your life change without changing something. There is a big difference between wanting your life to change and changing it. Is life something that happens to you or do you happen to it?

The Cornerstones are not something that you apply to your existing life, they are the foundation of a new one.

Always keep in mind the new paradigm. Visualize that new person you've decided you really want to be. Having done that, you are already on your way and everything else will fall in into place. Your new priorities will be set and you will live your life accordingly.

Don't be afraid to re-evaluate your paradigm frequently. If you aren't clear where you are headed, you aren't likely to get there. If you are clear about what it is you seek, but still have difficulties making progress, it will be your old paradigm holding you back. Excuses will inevitably come from the old paradigm. The old rules only apply if you allow them to. Remember the saying, "If an excuse is good enough, it becomes a reason."

The Effect on Others

Realize that others around you might not be as thrilled with your new paradigm and lifestyle. It will cause changes in them as well—changes that they may not welcome. However, anyone who genuinely cares about you will ultimately see the value in what you are doing.

Children will imitate the behavior of their parents. Think about whether you would prefer to have them copy your old habits, or your new ones. They may not always be thrilled to have to wait while you complete an agreement before attending to their requests, but in the end, you will be giving them something much greater.

Spouses will typically feel threatened. They may fear being left behind. They may not welcome the attention that you get as you become more alive and happy. But this is your life, and anyone who loves you should be able to accept that. After some rocky moments, things will settle down and the new routines will become as comfortable as the old routines.

Friends might feel estranged. You've altered these relationships as well. You may find your tolerance lessening for people who don't do what they say. They may not like you as well either, particularly if your progress makes them more aware of their own shortcomings. I can't say that I lost the friends that I had when I was fat; I still keep in contact with them, but they are not a big part of my life anymore. They've ultimately come to accept who I am but we have much less in common now and less reason to see each other. Instead, I've met many new people doing the things that I've learned in the Cornerstones.

These new friendships provide support for my new paradigm the same way that the old friendships provided support for the old paradigm.

And let's not forget co-workers and bosses that may not be so happy to see you disturbing *their* universe. Even the slightest change can be viewed as a big threat in the workplace, even if it doesn't appear to be job related. You are going to have a different set of priorities and they may not always fit quite as well your old ones did.

About a year after becoming comfortable with the Cornerstones, I left my old job to work as a consultant in the computer industry—something that I really wanted to do, and something that was part of my new paradigm. I didn't realize how much my old relationships were holding me back until I was surrounded by people who didn't know me any other way. I found myself developing friendships with people that I met as I worked on the Cornerstones, people who were already doing the things that I was learning. I became friends with runners, massage therapists, and yoga instructors. I met people into meditation, health foods, and journal keeping. Part of the thrill of the Cornerstones is having new relationships form and allowing new ideas into your life. These people all helped to validate my new way of thinking and I had less trouble abandoning my old ways.

When Dr. Bradley teaches his course on the Cornerstones, he has people pair up into "support buddies" and make agreements with each other. Others have formed support groups. This is one point that I disagree with him on. Frequently, I see the "buddies" supporting each other more in failure than in success. When one is successful and the other isn't, it tends to drag the successful one back to the old ways.

When I originally took the class, I think that I was actually fortunate in a sense because my "buddy" quit after the first class. Rather than finding a replacement, I just worked on making agreements with myself. I made myself my *own* support buddy. I learned to rely on myself rather than making commitments to another person. Who could possibly be more important than myself in making a commitment?

If you feel you need support, find people that are part of your new paradigm rather than your old one.

The Butterfly Technique

As you develop each of the four Cornerstones, it is important to take on new challenges in your agreements. You must continually push the boundaries of each Cornerstone a little further out as you gain strength. To attempt to take on too much too quickly is, of course, a serious mistake. It will lead rapidly to discouragement and disappointment with broken agreements and further enforce a self-image of failure.

On the other hand, not trying to find new limits and develop new interests will result in little or no change in your life. Keep in mind that you are changing your life, not waiting for your life to change. You are not simply applying something to your life like a diet or a pill and expecting results. You are actively recreating yourself in the role that you truly want to play. You are examining every aspect of your life and deciding whether it belongs in your new life or not. And I mean every aspect, not only the ones that you feel directly deal with your fat. Fat is a symptom, not a disease. There is no value in treating the fat, only in correcting the underlying life.

I found a simple technique that I think of as the Butterfly Technique, to guide me into new territories. When I am questioning myself about what new tasks and goals to take on, I try to tune into that little flutter in my stomach that we commonly refer to as having butterflies.

I've learned to use those butterflies as kind of a compass to point to new areas and directions worth pursuing. As I ponder what new paths to take and what agreements to make along the way, I try to stop and reflect on what the butterflies are telling me.

If I think about something and I feel nothing in my stomach, it probably isn't a challenging enough endeavor. More than likely it is way too easy for me and would serve no developmental purpose. Possibly, it might be something that I have no genuine interest in, something that I think I just "should" do, but can't really envision myself attempting.

On the other hand, if I think about something and feel gripping fear in my stomach that feels more like some kind of pre-historic pterodactyls than butterflies, I know it may be something to think about down the road but it isn't something that I can handle right now.

The ideal feeling is just a slight flutter, one that represents a tiny bit of fear mixed with a tiny bit of excitement—something that I'm not sure I could accomplish but would feel good if I did, and something that if I were to attempt and fail, wouldn't be the end of the world. Moreover, if I did fail, the failure might give me some new ideas about how to proceed in the future.

I believe that those little butterflies serve a tremendously useful purpose in managing our lives. Most of us probably have come to believe that feeling a little nervous is not a good thing and we avoid it. I think that it is more than a coincidence that those butterflies live in the same place that we associate with food—our stomachs. Food is soothing and certainly can help drown out the flutters of the butterflies, especially if our stomachs are packed to the limit leaving no room for the butterflies to fly at all.

Unfortunately, avoiding all nervousness eventually leads us into boring, predictable lives. The thrill that we used to experience when we were young and taking on a new activity is forgotten as we settle into our adult lives. We strive for banality and routine and then wonder why we become miserable, bored, and frustrated with life. Why? Whose idea was that? Where do we pick up the notion that at some age we should stop developing?

A small percentage of the population manages not to think that way. I have met people well into their 80's training for a marathon, learning yoga, learning a foreign language, writing a journal, and traveling to distant places like Africa. They are as vital and interesting as any younger person is. Somehow, they have managed to continue to seek out new areas of life and have never gotten out of the habit of developing themselves. They approach life with the same zest that a teenager has preparing for a first prom, or that a bride-to-be approaches her wedding.

These people do not have some genetic difference. These people have cultivated a habit that most of us once had and lost—curiosity. They've learned to trust their butterflies and to treat life as a journey, not a destination. They don't allow themselves to live inside a prison of fear, waiting for their lives to get better. They don't see life as something that happens to them; it is something that they create.

This is the approach that you must take as you learn about the Cornerstones. Always continue to picture yourself in some slightly new role doing something just a little more difficult than you had previously imagined. Learn to welcome the butterflies, not avoid them.

Certainly, I'm not advocating living with constant nervousness. But, if you realize that you haven't been visited by the butterflies in quite a while, maybe once a month, it is time to seek them out.

The Cornerstones have lead me into so many areas that I never would have even considered in my fat days. I have traveled to unusual places like Africa and India. I have struggled with learning Spanish and experienced the thrill of being understood (if only a little bit) in the middle of Mexico and Costa Rica. I have managed to sit at a piano and play Ragtime music, which I always loved listening to, but had never dared to envision myself actually playing. And, I found myself crossing the finish line of the New York City Marathon having once thought anybody who even owned a pair of running shoes was a fool.

Acquire a Taste for Adventure!

My description of each Cornerstone is meant only to be a starting point. Each Cornerstone is a subject area that you could pursue at great length on its own. I have outlined the general concepts and added some of my own experiences as well as some from people I have met teaching the Cornerstones. Where possible, I have included references to other sources that further describe a particular Cornerstone to keep you going. But ultimately, the decision is really all yours. Exactly how you accomplish your goal needs to come from you and be yours alone. There never can be a magic formula that will handle every individual's life and personality; it has to be created by everybody for themselves.

Take a few chances! What do you really have to lose?

Suggestions

- Make your most difficult Cornerstone part of your morning routine and it will become a habit.

- Watch for warning signs when one of the Cornerstones starts to become more difficult.

- Always evaluate your Cornerstones in your journal at the end of each day. Use the template at the back of this book as a guideline for your journal format.

- Make an agreement within each Cornerstone every day.

- Forget about living life on a weekly basis. If you slip, just keep going. There is no beginning and there is no ending, just a continuous process of living.

- Think of the Cornerstones in the context of the new you, not just tasks that you are adding to your old life.

- Look for support by finding people that are already part of your new paradigm, not your old.

- Remember the Butterfly Technique.

- Acquire a taste for adventure!

Favorite Excuses

- I only use the Cornerstones that are easy for me.

- Once I get thin, I'll be able to do all of the Cornerstones.

- It isn't necessary to track my Cornerstones in the journal; I can remember how I'm doing.

- I'm going to start really working on that Cornerstone next Monday.

- I think I'll wait until after the holidays or vacation or whenever to start doing the Cornerstones.

Add your favorite excuses here!

- _____
- _____
- _____
- _____
- _____
- _____
- _____
- _____
- _____
- _____
- _____
- _____

4

Cornerstone I: Journaling

The Good Old Days

I hope that you had a chance to watch *The Civil War* series on PBS a few years ago. It was broadcast every night for a week, and I believe the total time for the documentary was about 11 hours.

The series had received such tremendous reviews that I was curious about it even though I knew that I wouldn't have the time available to sit down every night for 2 or 3 hours. Instead, I videotaped the entire series, planning to watch it slowly, bit by bit, as I had the time.

I thought I'd begin watching just a few minutes of the series one Saturday morning as I was doing some laundry. I figured I'd just make a dent in viewing the 11 hours and then get on with the other activities that I had planned for that day. But, as I watched the show, I became so engrossed in the story, that I couldn't stop watching. Rather than watch the 30 minutes or so that I'd planned, I found myself watching the entire series straight through, all 11 hours at once! It was so captivating that I just couldn't shut it off. I popped tape after tape into the machine, anxious to continue with the next segment.

The next day I was thinking about my reaction to the documentary. What in the world had been so captivating about 11 hours of Civil War history? I certainly already knew the story line, there were no cliffhangers, and the South still didn't win! The episodes were made up mostly of old, black and white photographs interspersed with interviews with historians. Frankly, I'd never even paid much attention to the Civil War before, but something had brought that period of history to life in a way that I'd never experienced before, not in 8th grade history, and not even in *Gone With the Wind.*

What I eventually realized had made the series so unusual was the fact that much of the narration had been taken verbatim from the diaries and journals of the people living at that time. Rather than simply illustrate history with voice-over narration and explanation, the documentary makers chose passages from the diaries of the soldiers, generals, politicians, and civilians who were living at the time, and read them as if they were happening in "real time". This brought the story to life in a way that was very, very different from anything that I'd experienced before.

What I had assumed I would see was analysis and information—the equivalent of a history teacher dragging us through dates and events. What I got instead turned out to be much more. I was treated to the *thoughts and feelings* of the participants when they didn't know what tomorrow would bring. I was exposed to the thinking of people who had to decide what they would do next, possibly risking their lives and their families' futures, and literally be ready to die.

The series contained the gripping entries of a soldier wondering to himself in his diary if he would ever see his wife and children again, as he waited sleeplessly the night before a big battle; the hidden fears and insecurities of generals who had to make history changing decisions, sending people to their deaths while keeping a brave face for the troops; the grief of a mother who had to raise her children alone now that she had received news of her husband's death. All of these people recorded their thoughts in their journals.

Instead of happening in the past tense in traditional documentary style, much of the show was presented in present tense. We were able to get into the heads of the people that were there, read their thoughts and feel their feelings. These people all turned to their journals to express themselves—to get "in touch" with themselves—while working through their lives and the decisions that they were faced with.

I realized that these were real people with the same fears and frustrations that I deal with everyday—okay, maybe a little more than I deal with—but I still felt a connection that hadn't been there before, something beyond the facts and dates that I'd heard before.

What struck me as even more strange, the more I thought about it, was the fact that the documentary makers seemed to have so many journals to choose from. It wasn't just Abraham Lincoln and Robert E. Lee that you might think of making notes for historians in later generations. It was also the "little people"—people with terrible penmanship and poor grammar and spelling skills. People who had every reason in the world to be doing something else took time out of their lives to sit down with a journal in the evening. Even tough soldiers in the field who I would have thought of as too "macho" to do anything as ridiculous as carry a diary with them into war, used their journals to sort themselves out.

Apparently, there was a time in history when journal keeping was as common as sitting down to watch television in the evenings is today. This was a time when nobody felt silly making an effort to understand themselves, when taking the time to *reflect on life* made as much sense as watching some foolish sitcom on television to *escape it* does now.

The Daily Struggle

Journal Keeping is one of the Four Cornerstones, and it is the first Cornerstone to learn because it will be used as a springboard to the other three. Many people have trouble with the idea of keeping a journal when they first encounter the concept. I was one of them.

At first, I could barely write even a single sentence. The workbook that we used only had room for about a paragraph each day and I never could fill it. I would sit and struggle to produce even the most simple sentence. However, I believe my first agreement in the course was that I would write "something" every day. It didn't have to be long and it didn't have to amount to much, but that no matter what, I would sit down every evening and write.

I got in the habit of pulling out my journal while I watched television. I would just sort of jot something down during commercial breaks. Usually, just a line or two about what had happened that day was all that I could manage.

I couldn't imagine that anything in my life was worth putting on paper. I was appalled at how pathetic it looked on the page. My penmanship is beyond legibility most of the time, even to myself. My sentences were incomplete and my spelling was atrocious. At first I thought, "My God, what if somebody sees this?" But then I realized that it made so little sense and was so illegible that there was little risk of anybody taking much of an interest in what I'd written. There certainly was nothing going on in my life worth keeping a secret; it wasn't even worth writing about.

But somehow, in the 6 weeks that the course lasted, I managed to write a tiny bit each day. At first, it took conscious planning to schedule exactly when I would keep my journaling agreement. I had to fight with myself to renew the agreement each day. But, after a week or two, it just became part of the evening activities. Very quickly, the power of the daily agreement would take over. Before making the agreement, I would debate and agonize over whether this was such a good idea anymore, but once I said, "I agree to write in my journal tonight at 7:00", I felt a huge weight lift from me. The discussion was over, the deal was struck. I wasn't worrying about tomorrow and today was decided. My body started to listen to my mind and follow instructions. All of the energy that I was expending on debating with myself was now free for other things, and at 7:00, I would simply execute the agreement.

I rarely wrote anything of value or significance. My first entry consisted only of four lines. Here it is (I've done my best to decipher the penmanship and have corrected the spelling errors):

> *It was a fairly productive day, but a washout as far as eating. I was tired from going out with Tommy last night. Joe is apparently going to resign today or tomorrow. I enjoyed the first class.*

Hardly the stuff of a future PBS documentary. At least I didn't write about the weather (that came the next day). I had no visions of great grandchildren pouring over my prose with intense curiosity. However, at the time, I would have died if anybody had seen what I'd written. I kept my journal hidden from my wife. In fact, only in writing this, 20 years later, have I gone back to read it. Only now would I begin to have the courage to let someone else see what I'd written. At the time, that entry was the equivalent of pouring my heart out. It was as "in touch" with myself as I could get.

The workbook we used in the class for our journal had space for only about a dozen short sentences. By the end of the first week, I was usually able to come up with about 10 sentences each day. They were similar to what I'd written the first day—just the bare minimum of what had happened to me.

But about a week into the journaling, I had a terribly frustrating day. Even the vague details would fill more than the small space we had allotted in the workbook. So, I continued on a second sheet. When I read that entry now, I realize that I needed somebody to talk to, some way of unloading my frustrations. At a point when I would typically have turned to the refrigerator for solace, I found that I had a new tool—my journal.

I didn't realize it then, but I was starting to use the journal to do more than record my actions. Most of that entry dealt with the details of my frustrating job situation and the specifics of the project I was working on, but I concluded with something different:

> *I'm tired of being taken for granted. If only I knew what to do as an alternative. I do like the work, just not the environment.*

I asked myself if possibly I shouldn't look for a new line of work. It sounds trivial, but a subtle shift was beginning to occur. I was dealing with feelings and alternatives, not just facts. The idea had popped out and I hadn't really known it was there. Instead of getting lost in an out-of-control binge, I had some new information to ponder. Something inside me was beginning to speak up, and it wasn't just an escape fantasy. I was thinking about what I wanted in realistic terms—a new environment, not a new career.

Within a few weeks, journaling became quite automatic. Seeing the pages filled from previous days gave me a sense of power and satisfaction. I never bothered to go back and read them; I'm not sure I could have anyway. But there they were, day after day of senseless scribbles, and I began to feel very good about it. I even began to look forward to it!

I do remember one evening when some unexpected disaster came along at work and I didn't get home until after 2:00 a.m. My routine was disrupted and it was already way past time to get to bed. I had forgotten my journal agreement completely. By that time, I had gotten good enough at it that I didn't agree that I would write at a specific time anymore, just that I would write each night. I was already sound asleep when, for some unknown reason, I woke up and snapped to attention. I looked at the clock and it was about 3:00 a.m. Something was wrong. My journal! I got out of bed, got the journal out, and wrote next to nothing, but at least I'd kept the agreement. I went back to bed and felt a deep satisfaction that I was indeed becoming somebody that I could count on, even when the world seemed to conspire to thwart my efforts.

Building a Relationship with a Journal

My journal keeping became a welcomed task. It was like a conversation with a very close friend. I began to trust myself more and open up to it. This was all very similar to the path that any relationship follows. Tentative at first, testing the water, then opening up more and more as the trust builds. My journal didn't judge me, it just listened to my feelings and was there whenever I needed it.

Another interesting moment came one day when something particularly upsetting happened at work. The director had come by and chewed out a co-worker. I couldn't help overhearing the conversation. I was aware of the real situation and felt that the co-worker was being treated unfairly. I remember sitting at my desk, not knowing quite what to do with all of the anger and frustration I was feeling. Without realizing what I was doing, I started writing down my feelings on a pad of paper. I had filled a whole page before I realized that I was journaling. My feelings were intense enough that I couldn't wait until that evening to "talk" through them with my journal. Just putting my thoughts down on paper, no matter how irrational or rambling they might be, made me feel so much better. I folded the papers up and stuck them in my pocket to tuck into my journal when I got home that night.

In the past, when something disturbing happened, I would quietly slip off to my favorite vending machine and push the feelings away with candy bars. It was as if I would swallow emotions back down inside me. I didn't want to even have feelings—certainly not upsetting ones—but really any feelings. I was as apt to "eat" good feelings as well as uncomfortable ones. Somehow, the whole idea of experiencing an emotion frightened me.

The journal began to let me safely experience feelings bit by bit. Just putting them on the page seemed to get them out of my system, which of course I wanted to do. I still wasn't that eager actually to experience them, but somehow just putting them on paper let me see them for what they were and I could begin to free myself from the fear and think about what was going on in a more rational way.

When I had filled up the workbook and Dr. Bradley's class was over, I still wasn't sure how committed I was to this journaling idea, but I was sure I wanted to continue for a while longer. I went to an office supply store and bought a small blank record book. I didn't want to buy a traditional diary. I thought that looking at a whole year's worth of blank pages might discourage me more than help. On a day-to-day basis, I liked the journal, but I still wasn't sure that I could commit to an entire year. The little record book had enough paper to last about a month. I continued writing in the same format as the workbook had outlined.

I filled the small book and then tried buying a slightly larger one. I still chose one that was completely blank. I wanted to write in the date as well as the text so I could renew my agreement daily, rather than feel obligated by a pre-printed date on each page. I suppose this sounds trivial, but I wanted the commitment to come from inside me, not from an external source. It was my life and I was determined to seize control of it.

The idea about switching jobs continued with more in depth entries. I probed my feelings for clues about what it was that I was seeking. I didn't simply look for a different job; I developed my needs through the journal. I realized that I wanted to be an independent consultant, not just another employee. It was a dream that I barely knew that I had. I took my time and prepared myself, sought out new information, and processed it in my journal.

Strange New World

After about a year of using all of the Cornerstones, I felt secure enough to take on a new level of living. I had lost a lot of weight and really recreated myself. It wasn't that I was "finished" at all, I never would be, I had just adopted a whole new way of life and it was beginning to bear fruit. I finally moved towards my newly identified goal: I ventured out into the world of self-employment.

What I noticed first was that people who hadn't known me before treated me differently than I was used to. I received more respect. None of them seemed to have any idea that I had been much fatter. Why would they? I carried myself with more confidence. When I said something, people listened, not just out of courtesy, but with a different level of attention.

That wasn't all as wonderful as it might sound. It was actually quite frightening. Having spent the better part of 30 years being essentially invisible and then suddenly becoming visible, was more than a little alarming. My sarcastic humor that nobody had paid much attention to before could now cut deeply. I had to learn to back off and adjust my level of intensity.

Every night I recorded my new experiences in the journal. It wasn't as if I instantly felt better when I wrote, but I never turned to food to wash away my fear. I just kept working each of the Cornerstones, taking step after step, day after day, and recording it all in my journal.

The little things that I hadn't noticed before really seemed the most disturbing—riding in an elevator, for example. When I was obese, people would stand much further away from me. Now, they thought nothing of standing right next to me, even touching me occasionally. It felt strange and uncomfortable.

Another example might happen at a grocery store while I was standing in the aisle choosing a product. I had never realized how people instinctively would move away from me when I was fat rather than stand close to me. Now they didn't, and it was disturbing. At first I was never sure what was different, I just felt that something wasn't right. I used my journal to seek out the difference and bring it into my consciousness.

On the subway, I was used to having the seat next to me be the last one taken. Now, nobody seemed to think twice about sitting next to me. If fact, I remember one day a very attractive woman plunked herself down right next to me when there were plenty of other seats available. Not only that, but she started talking to me! Something seemed so odd and I felt terribly awkward. Then I realized—she was flirting with me! I didn't have a clue how to handle that. I had absolutely no experience with such things. Nothing in my past prepared me for this moment. I felt incredibly foolish and once again turned to my journal to sort out what had happened.

Women especially seem to have more trouble when they lose weight and become more physically attractive. Men, traditionally the aggressors, may come from everywhere with an intensity that she may never have experienced before. If a female has been overweight her entire life, she may never have developed the coping skills necessary to handle men. She could easily be defenseless at a time when defenses are most important, and it is not unusual to see somebody regain all of the weight to re-introduce a barrier to the world. Everything that sounded so wonderful in a daydream might turn out to be quite terrifying when actually experienced.

The journal functions as a pressure relief valve if used correctly. It provides a way to vent frustration productively and lay out new plans based on the mistakes that are made daily.

Over the years, my journaling improved. I spent much more time just emoting rather than detailing events. I would start by putting down the bare essentials of the day, and then flush things out with my feelings about the events.

I worked toward what is known as a *stream of consciousness*. I made no effort to write with any particular structure. I didn't bother much with paragraphs or complete sentences. I just plugged the pen into my feelings and let it flow, essentially bypassing my intellect. I never had any idea what would come out when I would sit down to write. It was usually a surprise and frequently I found myself revealing things about myself that surprised me. I learned how intuitive I was, and how frequently I knew exactly what was going to happen before it did.

Problems sometimes seemed to correct themselves. I rarely made myself come up with a solution as I wrote. I just spit the problem out and put it down on paper. If I was doing some self-destructive thing on a regular basis, I found that by being honest and not hiding my behavior, I would almost seem to correct the problem automatically. It was if just writing about it somehow relieved me of the issue.

I made regular agreements and wrote about the outcome. I focused my agreements on what I wanted to be doing, not so much on what I wanted to stop doing. If an agreement was poorly thought out, it usually revealed its flaws when I wrote it down. If I broke the agreement in a particular way, the pattern would become apparent as I wrote about it in the journal. I would then rework the agreement in a more rigorous way. Somehow, writing about the ways I would break an agreement prevented me from using that approach too many times. It was as if writing sent the whole process through a different part of my brain and let me treat it more intelligently and deal with it rationally.

I could think about a situation forever, but I never could do much about it until I wrote it down. I began to accept problems as an ongoing reality. I got away from that "beginning" and "end" mentality that I had before. I learned that whatever frustration I was dealing with would eventually be straightened out, and then inevitably a completely new one would come along. Instead of trying to ignore or avoid my frustrations, I learned how to work through them. At least I'd get some new problems to deal with, rather than being stuck with the same old ones over and over.

I kept seeking out bigger and bigger journals. What had started out as a trickle became a flood of words each day. I got tired of running to the office supply store each month and finally started buying books big enough to hold an entire year's writing. Instead of fearing all of those blank pages, I would begin to look at them with excitement and wonder what would get written on them. I knew that they would hold the story of my life, inside and out, and I was starting truly to think that I had a life worth living and one worth writing about.

I reached a point where I had to special order the largest blank book available. None of the standard ones stocked were large enough to support my "habit". I can't help being amused every year when I order that book. The look on the clerk's face is priceless. He can't imagine why one of the many styles that they already stock wouldn't suit my needs.

I almost never looked back at my entries. In later years, I would sometimes spend the year-end holidays randomly reading passages from the previous year, not necessarily looking for special events. When something major did happen, it would somehow intrigue me to read what I had been thinking about before it happened—when I was unsuspecting and had no idea what was waiting around the corner.

The last couple of years I started writing a year-end summary. Not by looking at past writings, but just by sitting down and seeing what came back to me from the previous year. With a year's passage, tiny insignificant moments tend to come together into a much bigger and more interesting story. Patterns and trends were much more obvious. I would frequently find that major changes in my thinking had actually been building in small ways that went unnoticed at the time. An off-hand comment, a dream, or a random event would frequently start a chain reaction that was quite fascinating.

After 20 years of journaling, I have generated quite a stack of books. It is strange to look at them now. They sit quietly on the shelf like any other book, but inside those books the pages are filled with my thoughts at the time of the birth of my children—what I was thinking before, during, and after. They contain all of the thrills and all of the pain of being a parent. The pages are filled with the dissolution of my marriage and all of the pain and introspection that came with it. And the pages chronicle my trials and tribulations of being single and doing it as a person who now has the tools to take on just about any task imaginable.

I still don't let anyone see them. There are definitely things in those books that would ruin any chance I might ever have of being appointed to the Supreme Court, should some congressional committee ever subpoena my journals. But what the hell, it's all me, warts and all. If I ever do get the desire to run for public office, a paper shredder should clean up my record, just like the "pros"!

I only wish I had the journals that would have been written in the first 30 years of my life, had I known about this technique. Things that seemed unbearably painful when I was 10 years old, might reveal an awful lot now.

A Never Ending Story

I don't mean to write about the journal process too much in the past tense. This is all stuff that I still do on a daily basis and plan to do until the end of my life. I can't imagine it any other way now. What seemed impossible to do in the beginning now seems impossible to do without. The weight loss wasn't an event that started and finished, it is something that happened as a byproduct of a new lifestyle. And it is a lifestyle that continues today and will continue tomorrow.

I experiment now with journaling at different times of the day. If I write in the evening, I tend to focus more on the facts of the day and my reactions. If I write in the morning, dreams are fresh and my emotions tend to be more accessible. I just tune into the emotion that I'm feeling, try to describe it, and leave it at that. Usually the source of the feeling will reveal itself in time.

I frequently switch my routine when it comes to journaling. When I'm looking for a new path in life, I tend to write in the morning. When I'm clearer about where I'm heading, I like to write in the evening and evaluate my progress. I wouldn't have been able to be that loose about my journaling in the beginning. I required the daily regimen and agreements to make room in my life for something new. But now, it is anything but a chore and I welcome it. I would have never believed that could happen in the beginning.

Doing It

I hesitate to talk too much about what I'm doing in my current Cornerstone efforts. People sometimes try to get there too fast and don't want to experience the growth from an initial effort that leads to more exciting things. All of the Cornerstones are very personal and they must grow out of your own desires. The journey is the adventure.

At a minimum, there are some journaling basics that I recommend for everyone. First of all, complete confidentiality is essential. Somehow, you must make yourself comfortable with what you write in your journal and that it is for you alone. Forget about later generations reading your journal. That is not its purpose and may not be at all desirable.

The value of the journal is in the writing, not in the reading. It makes no difference how well you write. You will get better as you write more, but that isn't the point. The process (not the result) is what is the most important.

A session with a journal is not unlike a session with a psychotherapist. Complete confidentiality is necessary or you will never feel comfortable getting to the root of your feelings. If necessary, develop code words for the things that are particularly uncomfortable. You will know what you mean and that is all that is important. If there is someone else that will be tempted to read what you write, you must take steps to protect yourself. If you feel too vulnerable with your writing, the beneficial effect will be lost.

Hiding your journal or keeping it at work is another possibility. If you leave it out in the open, someone will invariably read it. I met a woman in one of the workshops who felt so ashamed of her size that she cut all of the tags out of her clothing so that the housekeeper couldn't snoop in her closets and figure out her dress size. Imagine the vulnerability that this person felt with having a journal detailing her innermost thoughts. Finding a way to feel private is extremely important.

Lock it away somewhere, if necessary. Buy a desk or a cabinet with a locking drawer. There are all sorts of small, safe containers available that have combination locks or keys. Another alternative is to use computer software that can maintain and password protect a journal.

It probably isn't necessary to keep what you write, since the value is in the writing. If something is particularly disturbing, you might want to consider writing it and then destroying it. The point is to get it out, not necessarily to have it as a reference.

It is absolutely necessary to write, not just think. Many people try to "think" their journals. For some reason, and I really don't know why, that just doesn't work. It could be that the process of writing itself is a much higher brain function that simply thinking. Writing is a skill developed by human beings only in very recent times. It is possible that writing about your life tends to send the information through an entirely different section of your brain, which in turn affects your behavior. Obviously, we've all *thought* about our problems before, what we want is to begin to *deal* with them, and the act of writing seems to stimulate that process.

Pay attention to your resistance to writing. You probably will actually feel your body resisting change. Your inner self will come to know that this is serious business and it may not always welcome your probes into your sub-conscious. Sometimes, if you can't write about something, write about what you are experiencing as you resist writing. This can begin to unravel the mystery and it will at least continue to confirm your level of trust with yourself. You agreed to write, and you are writing.

Stream of Consciousness

Try to just flow with your words. This will feel very strange at first and quite nice later on. Take a moment to think about how you think. Most of us jump from thought to thought, sometimes on completely unrelated subjects. Our minds are a mish-mash of ideas, not necessarily a logical, continuous flow. The thoughts come and go and we may never again return to them. Other times, we might bring something up continuously. Different ideas come from everywhere and at any moment.

When you are journaling, imagine yourself plugging that pen into a faucet on the side of your head, turning it on, and then letting the thoughts just flow out without any further processing. It is as if you've opened a drain and let things empty out.

Don't spend much time, if any, analyzing what you are writing. Don't try to tidy things up like a script for a television show with neat endings and conclusions. Sherlock Holmes is not going to show up in the last few sentences of your journal entry and make it all make sense. Mysteries can go on forever in a journal. That is part of the experience.

The Journal is a Daily "Must"

No other Cornerstone is as important on a daily basis as keeping your journal. I recommend that you make a daily agreement within each Cornerstone, but it is an absolute "must" that you track everything in your journal each day.

Don't look at the Cornerstone concept as a program that you adopt and then drop when things get tough. It isn't something to pick back up again when you feel more "up to it". The tough times are as much a part of it as the good times. In fact, the tough times are almost *more* a part of it than the good times. Obviously, if our lives were all good, nobody would be reading this book. What we need is something for the bad times, to grab hold of them and make them ours so that they don't destroy our good intentions.

Those disaster days are exactly when you truly need your journal. Those are the days when you will reveal yourself most, when your inner self is trying to tell you something. Even days that appear to be a disaster for external reasons typically show themselves to be at least partly your own "doing" when examined in your journal.

Learn to look at disaster days as a wealth of clues to be examined and processed in your ongoing mystery of life management. There will certainly be red herrings, but not as many as you might think. Using your journal daily will begin to show you just how much of your life you really do control, and it will direct you in gaining control of the areas that you don't have control of now.

Binge Journaling

Focus on more than being fat and overeating. Remember that they are only symptoms. Look beyond those problems to the real issues. A good technique for doing this is to turn to your journal when you feel a binge coming on. Make an agreement that when you feel yourself losing control that you will give yourself 10 minutes to write in your journal before you continue with the binge. Don't make the binge the issue. Realize that the urge to eat is coming from something else, something that possibly happened earlier in the day and now your unconscious mind is trying to push it away. You aren't agreeing not to binge; you are simply inserting 10 minutes of journaling as part of the binge process. Don't fight the binge, roll with it.

If you try this, chances are you will find yourself staring at an empty page and feeling tremendous anger, or sadness, or frustration. I can just about guarantee that you won't be able to write. Your mind is trying desperately to turn off whatever it is feeling, not let it out. But if you sit there and tune into the feeling, the thoughts just might begin to flow. Try to identify which feeling (or feelings) you are experiencing. Fear? Sadness? Jealousy? Disappointment? Anger? Frustration? Or maybe you are feeling what we might think of as a positive emotion. Excited? Important? Triumphant? Loving? It is not unusual to have good things trigger a binge as well as bad things. Many of us work to undo accomplishments through binge eating. We feel as if we aren't worthy and set out to prove it. We want to believe that whatever good thing happened must have been a fluke!

The point of this exercise is not to fight off the binge. It is to steal a little information from it. To find out just what might be going on inside you. It will never be simple and it certainly won't clear itself up in one or two attempts. Binge eating is an act of self-destruction and it is unlikely that some simple solution is going to appear in your journal. It is even more likely that your inner-self will not want to participate in coping with this behavior and will do everything in its power to avoid revealing itself.

Over time, tiny bits of information will begin to add up to bigger things. When you are feeling the urge to binge, you may be less likely to resist revealing yourself. A tremendous amount of energy is being channeled into the binge, and in a way, your defenses are down. You just might learn something if you take 10 minutes to probe your thoughts.

Play a Game of Name That Emotion

Look at the Feeling Identification Prompt List at the back of the book when you find yourself unable to describe a feeling. Scan down the list until you find something that seems to fit your mood and then write that word in your journal. See if anything else begins to flow once you've identified your emotion.

It is quite possible that you are feeling more than one emotion. Write them all down. It can be tricky when feelings start to run together. Sorting them out is like trying to identify all of the spices used in a recipe, but if you learn to tune in, you will be able to detect just what you're feeling.

If you manage to identify your feelings, try to see what flows after that. What happened that day to lead to those feelings? Work backwards. When did you start being aware of the feeling? What time? Was it already with you when you woke up in the morning? Did it start when you got to work? Find associations, but don't spend much time drawing conclusions.

At other times, it may work better to start with the facts of the day and then see what feelings grow out of writing about them. However, I want to stress that there are no rules. There are no cookie cutter approaches to journaling. These are only suggestions to get you started. This is your life. Write about it anyway you see fit.

Awareness is all that we are after with the journal, and not just awareness of the bad times. It is quite possible that everything is going fine and you will want to be aware of that too. An awareness of feelings at all levels at all times is the ultimate goal.

Your Journal is Free Therapy

If you need any further motivation, think of your journal as a free session with a psychotherapist. It would cost you at least a $100 to tell all of that stuff to a shrink. So, whenever you write, consider yourself $100 richer!

However, I don't want you to think of your journal as a cure. It isn't something that you do until you get better and then stop. It is something that is now a part of your life, and it will eventually become a welcome part of it.

Your journal will serve as a path to the real you and it will serve you well as time goes by. You are never finished journaling unless you feel you are finished with life. And if you feel that you are finished with life, write about it.

The journal will make you aware of just who and what you are. This sounds so simple, but so few people have this awareness. We are bombarded with messages about who we "should" be from the day we are born. Our parents, friends, teachers, spouses, preachers, politicians, co-workers, bosses, children, and the media all have an idea of who we should be, and use every opportunity to tell us about it. How can we possibly avoid getting confused about what we really are? We rarely give ourselves any time to think about it, because it isn't really a part of our culture. The journal will at least let our own inner-self have an occasional moment to talk with us, and give us at least a shot at equal time in the midst of all of that confusion. Even the politicians have a law that guarantees them equal time. Why shouldn't we give ourselves the same consideration?

Suggestions

- For Your Eyes Only! Your journal is personal. Hide it, encode it, or do whatever is necessary to make yourself comfortable with the privacy of the contents.

- Write something everyday. It will become much easier with practice.

- Don't worry about penmanship, grammar, or spelling. Nobody is going to read your journal.

- Work towards a "Stream of Consciousness". The purpose is to get what you're feeling inside to the outside so you can deal with it.

- There is tremendous power in writing what you're feeling. Don't just think about it. Thinking can be just another way of not dealing with things.

- Start with what's going on in your life, but proceed from the facts to the feelings. Be honest about your emotions, especially if you don't like what you are feeling.

- Don't rush to draw conclusions. Just get to know yourself. Over time, your patterns will become more obvious.

- When you identify something you want to change, make agreements and write them down. Use the journal to analyze what happened. Proceed with harder (or easier) agreements.

- Experiment with writing in your journal at different (or multiple) times. Try writing when you feel an eating binge coming on. Delay the binge a few minutes and notice what feelings begin to surface.

- Use the Feelings List at the back of this book to tune into possible feelings that you are having, if you are stuck for something to write.

- Remember, this is FREE therapy!

- Acquire a taste for adventure!

Favorite Excuses

- Someone might read it.
- My penmanship is awful.
- My spelling is awful.
- My grammar is awful.
- I don't have the time.
- I can't think of anything to write.
- My life isn't interesting enough.
- I don't need to actually write, I can just think about what I would write.

Add your favorite excuses here!

- _____
- _____
- _____
- _____
- _____
- _____
- _____
- _____
- _____
- _____
- _____
- _____
- _____

5

Cornerstone II: Stress Reduction

The Trouble with Stress...

I wish I could begin by telling you about all of my wonderful accomplishments with Stress Reduction, the second Cornerstone. But frankly, if there is one Cornerstone that still causes me grief after all of these years, this is it.

For some this is the easiest Cornerstone, but for me there seems to be no end to my creativity when avoiding stress reduction. It is as if my body just doesn't want to give up feeling stressed; it is as if stress has become an addiction in itself.

In general, I think we tend to resist the Cornerstones that would help us the most. The part of our sub-conscious that doesn't want to change can be very clever in its ways of thwarting our efforts. Something about stress seems to make me not want to do anything about it, even though I'm usually quite aware of its presence.

I can see the effects of stress as it accumulates, chronicled daily in my journal. My general level of irritation increases and my patience decreases. I begin to crave less healthy foods. My resting pulse rate rises. I have difficulty sleeping. Concentration becomes difficult. I begin breaking agreements. I catch a cold, the flu, or some other illness.

As damaging as the effects of stress are, my resistance to reducing stress is always strong. In fact, the more I could benefit from some type of stress reduction, usually the more unappealing it becomes.

Even writing this section is by far the most difficult for me. My subconscious seems not to want to focus on the subject. The words won't flow and the sentences are awkward. My spelling has suddenly become abysmal. However, handling stress is extremely important because in so many ways stress is the undoing of our best intentions, and it is worthy of our constant attention.

Stress Reduction is by far the most abstract Cornerstone. Ironically, it can be the most pleasant and the most intriguing. I have met the most interesting people while pursuing stress reduction. I have made friends in areas of my life that just wouldn't have happened without my constant efforts to seek out new approaches to reducing stress.

Good Stress versus Bad Stress?

You might think as I got healthier and managed to get a handle on my life, that stress would automatically disappear. It is true that the type of stress has changed over the years. Twenty years ago, it seemed that the source of my stress was almost all the frustration from not doing what I wanted in life. My only stress reduction technique was overeating.

That kind of negative stress is still a part of my life from time to time, but I've also begun to experience a new kind of stress—positive stress. This is the stress generated from doing new things. It comes from the fears about facing new tasks and having new goals and intentions. Meeting new people and doing new things is every bit as stressful as avoiding them once was. Just because I am doing more of what I want in life doesn't mean that everything is easy.

I've begun to think of stress as neutral. There is little point in categorizing whether it is good or bad. It is just there; it is a by-product of living. It is similar to the heat generated by the friction from something moving. It may or may not be useful, but it will accumulate in us like any other waste product and it needs to be eliminated properly or it will cause even more problems.

Tired or Stressed?

Many people will describe themselves as tired after a day of work, but not many of us actually do physically exhausting things. Some people do, of course. Anybody who has a physically active job or chases after small children all day probably is genuinely tired, but for a lot of us what we are really feeling is stress.

Stress affects us much in the same way as being physically tired, so it is easy to get confused. In fact, the experts tell us that there are two different types of stress, physical and emotional, but the effects are the same.

I'm not sure that I ever really experienced physical stress until I started running long distances. While I trained for the marathon, I would find myself quite exhausted (as you might expect) and the effects were very similar to that caused by emotional stress. My body didn't seem to know the difference. I would snap at people, have trouble sleeping, and eat too much. If I had not known about the stress reduction techniques that I learned using the Cornerstones, I suspect that I would have abandoned my goal to complete a marathon.

Binge Eating as a Stress Reduction Technique

Whether or not they are aware of it, most people have some way of eliminating tension. For just about any fat person, overeating is the main approach to stress reduction. Fat people have found a very effective way of relieving tension. Unfortunately, their technique has some quite undesirable side effects. From the moment of our birth we are aware of how pleasant food can be and just about everyone turns to it in moments of stress. That includes both good and bad moments. We celebrate with food and we grieve with it.

As anyone reading this book realizes, overeating causes fat that in turn causes more stress. The fat helps us avoid new situations that are stressful, but it doesn't really solve anything, and it creates its own problems that "stress us out".

Obviously, binge eating is not a desirable approach to stress management. Many other better techniques can make a profound difference in your sense of well-being.

Stress Reduction in a Nutshell

In the chapter on journaling, we learned that we tend to eat our emotions. I believe that we also tend to eat our stress. This is one point where the interaction between the Cornerstones can be seen. We may have incorrectly learned that when we feel something we should "eat" that emotion away. We may also have learned that when we are tired or stressed we should attempt to "eat" that feeling away also. It would be almost impossible to determine what was driving an unhealthy desire to eat, and there really is no need to do so. If it is an emotion that requires expression, the journal will help. If it is stress accumulation, stress reduction will help. There is no point in worrying about the "why" of the situation; our daily attention to the Cornerstones will keep us on track. Too much self-analysis will result in "analysis paralysis", and little will be done to actually deal with the situation. If journaling and stress reduction are done on a routine daily basis, almost any problem will take care of itself, no matter what its source. Both Cornerstones will simultaneously provide tremendous value in coping with our lives.

There is a multitude of stress reduction techniques from which to choose. Here is a sampling:

- Meditation
- Relaxation Tapes
- Massage
- Yoga
- Dance
- Tai Chi
- Saunas
- Whirlpool or hot baths
- Deep Breathing
- Long, peaceful walks

Make an agreement to do something from the list everyday. You may need to make agreements just to learn about a technique, maybe to take a class or read a book, but do something about stress every day.

All of the techniques are quite fun, but I'll bet that no one reading this does any of them on a regular basis. Hopefully, something on the list will have some appeal to you even if it is something that you can't quite picture yourself doing at the moment.

One of the problems with the Stress Reduction Cornerstone versus the Journal Keeping Cornerstone is that many of the options tend to be a more "public". Writing in a journal should be very private, but attending a yoga class or dancing is a very public activity. Fat people generally don't like to try new things in front of other people and feel a sense of shame for even attempting something outside of their paradigm.

Fortunately, some of the choices are also private and can be accomplished without the knowledge of anyone. Mediation, a hot bath, or simply 10 minutes of deep, quiet breathing require no help from anyone else.

As you become more proficient at stress reduction and more courageous in general, some of the other options on the list may take on a new appeal. The trick is always to strike a balance between routine and adventure. I've known some people to listen to the same relaxation tape, day in and day out, for weeks and weeks. Establishing a routine is very important, but self-torture is unnecessary. When something starts to get dull, seek out a new approach.

My Evolving Battle with Stress

When I first learned about stress reduction, the only options Dr. Bradley mentioned were yoga, massage, meditation, and dance. There was no way I was going to waddle around in public trying to learn how to dance, nor was I at all interested in contorting my body like a pretzel in a yoga class when I could barely bend over to tie my shoes. And, as wonderful as the idea of a massage sounded, there was no way I was going to let anybody see my body let alone touch it!

That pretty much left meditation. Images came to my mind of gurus with shaved heads, white robes, and flowers, chanting mindlessly. I wasn't so sure about that either. The last thing I wanted was to be brainwashed and wind up at the airport trying to recruit new followers.

I came to realize that there is nothing magical or satanic about meditation. It is merely taking some quiet time, clearing the mind, and letting thoughts bubble up from the depths of our psyche.

I sought out various books on the subject and it turned out there are quite a few. They range from the very spiritual to the very clinical. *The Relaxation Response* by Herbert Benson seemed to be the all around best on the subject. He does a nice job of simplifying and de-mystifying meditation. He explains the why and the how in quite accessible terms and does a very good job at convincing the reader of the value of meditation.

Meditation comes down to a very simple concept—using either a nonsense or spiritual phrase repeatedly to clear the mind. Benson recommends sitting quietly and comfortably, focusing on your breath, and using the word "one" silently as you exhale. He talks about adopting a "passive" attitude and simply letting thoughts that enter your mind float away rather than pursue them. The goal is to let your mind shut down for some period of time, to let loose of all of your troubles, and to essentially clear your mind like you are erasing a blackboard. This process should continue for 10 to 20 minutes every day.

When I started, I never got even that elaborate. I simply made an agreement that as soon as I came home in the evening, I would lie down quietly for 10 minutes. During that time, I would do my best to clear my mind, and if I succeeded in shutting down my worries at all, I would begin to visualize myself as I had decided I wanted to be. I tried to create visual images of how I would look and what I would be doing in my new paradigm. Some days this was easy and others it was all but impossible.

I never got very good at the true meditation techniques. My mind was always quite stubborn, but it didn't seem to matter, the effect was there and gradually I became a little more comfortable with the idea.

Years later, I did attend several different classes on meditation. Strangely, I found that if I was with a group and we were all quietly meditating, my mind could go much deeper into itself and I came much closer to experiencing the things that the experts profess.

Even so, I never was able to bring the concepts home with me and achieve that level of success on my own. I suppose there were just too many distractions nearby begging for my attention. No matter how empty I succeeded in getting my mind, outside sounds would creep in—the sound of bills waiting to paid, the sound of the lawn growing outside needing cutting, etc. And strongest of all of course, was the call of the food in the refrigerator, seeping into my deepest thoughts…

But I did it every day. Just by giving myself 10 minutes completely to myself was very powerful. Spending even a minute focused and visualizing my new paradigm helped to make it into a reality, even though at the time that I was doing this it seemed almost worthless. But somehow just allowing those images into my mind, if only in the form of a fantasy, started things happening.

If you are curious about meditation, there is no limit to the directions you can take. You can pursue something like Transcendental Meditation and be given a secret mantra to chant that is chosen just for you. There are semi-religious groups that offer group meditation with a spiritual flair, and there are others like the Silva Mind Control organization that teach similar concepts in a more clinical way. But don't overlook just spending some time alone with yourself and doing nothing but thinking about where you want to go with your life. Anything is quite powerful in reducing the level of stress and keeping tabs on your new priorities.

As I became more comfortable with the idea of taking some time each day for stress reduction, I tried other approaches. I found that bookstores had a nice selection of guided imagery audio tapes. They ranged from general relaxation to specific topics. I stayed away from the weight loss specific tapes; I didn't want to confuse stress reduction with trying to get rid of fat even though they are quite related. I wanted this to be all mine and I didn't want to make stress reduction something I used to bring new rules into my life. Instead, I preferred the more general types of recordings, the ones with soothing music and perhaps a voice gently talking the listener into a deeper and deeper state of relaxation. Some of the more interesting tapes used only music and sound effects like the ocean waves, or a gentle rainstorm. Others were just an ambient, unstructured style of music that let my mind cut loose from its concerns.

I built up a collection of different tapes to keep things interesting. I found that if I heard the same tape too often, I would start to ignore it and go on worrying about life.

I did notice that the more stressed out I felt, the more excuses I found not to take time for stress reduction. My mind seemed to rebel against letting go of its frustrations. I would badly want to binge to get rid of the stress rather than just relax and let it dissipate on its own. But I stuck to it, and slowly the effects started to accumulate and my level of stress began to decline.

Massage

From the first night of the Cornerstone class, I was curious about massage. Something about the thought of just relaxing while somebody worked the stress away was very appealing. It was also very frightening.

I realized that I never liked anybody to touch me. To touch me meant that I had a body and I had worked so hard to detach my body from my mind that I wanted no reminders that that wasn't really the case.

As I wrote about my feelings in my journal, I came to realize that I hated all things that involved someone focusing on my body. Getting a haircut, seeing a doctor or a dentist, even having my eyes examined bothered me, once I thought about it. To be the object of someone else's attention made me feel tremendously self-conscious. So, the idea of lying down for an hour and letting somebody work over my body, well, that was just out of the question! Yet, somewhere inside of me there was a tingly little feeling that said, well maybe...

As my fat began to disappear, I began to be a little less self-conscious and felt a little more like I might like to try something like massage. I didn't make an agreement to get a massage. That would have been too big of a step. I just made an agreement to *find out* more about massage.

My execution of the agreement turned out to be somewhat humorous. My first stop, as usual, was the bookstore. I bought a nice big book on massage. It explained all of the wonderful "how's and why's" of a massage. It had great color pictures of different techniques and of loving couples in a state of bliss as they helped each other relax with various massage strokes, looking lovingly into each other's eyes.

But, other than some wishful thinking, the book didn't do me much good. I was married at the time and we had two small children. Stress was as much a part of our household as air. My innocent request to my wife that she try out some of the strokes shown on me didn't produce the same loving look that the woman pictured in the book had. Somehow, the images in the book just didn't map to reality. I realized that I was pretty much on my own with this one. Unfortunately, massage is just one of those things that require help from another person.

The only place I could think of to locate a massage therapist was in the Yellow Pages. Sure enough, there were many, many pages of listings for massage therapists. However, as I read the ads, I began to suspect that maybe they weren't quite as concerned with stress reduction as I was.

Ads that touted 7 day 24 hour service with "discretion assured" made me a little suspicious. Massage therapists that seemed to go only by their first name, usually something like Desiree or Bambi, and restricted their practice only to men, made me think that possibly I was headed in the wrong direction.

I guess I'll never know if the "House of Coeds" or the "Pussycat Massage Parlor" specializing in the "purrfect hands" were quite as legitimate as they claimed to be, because I decided that I'd already kept my agreement. I had researched how to find a massage and that was good enough. Nevertheless, the curiosity still lingered. Surely there was a source of legitimate massage somewhere. I was clear on my intentions, but the ways and means eluded me.

Then, one of the stranger moments in my Cornerstone pursuits happened. I was summoned for jury duty. I dreaded the thought. By this time, I was self-employed, having left my old unfulfilling job and started working as a self-employed consultant. That had worked out well, but now something like jury duty was a disaster. I had no benefits and that meant no jury duty pay from an employer. The $25 a day that the court was going to give me wasn't really going to make a dent in my living expenses.

I watched in dread as the judge shot down excuse after excuse from people trying to escape their requirement to serve on a jury. I knew that my excuses didn't come close to the ones that I had heard being offered, so I settled in and accepted my misfortune.

As I sat and listened to the other jurors being interviewed, I heard the woman sitting next to me announce her occupation as a licensed massage therapist. Her name wasn't anything like Bambi, it was simply Beth and she appeared to be quite normal. I guess I figured that if she weren't a legitimate therapist, she probably wouldn't be announcing that fact in the middle of the judicial system.

We were both chosen as jurors and the trial dragged on over the next week. We weren't allowed to discuss the trial until we began deliberations, so I spent the breaks and lunches talking with Beth to find out all that I could about massage.

She told me about her frustrations finding clients. The image of massage had become so warped by the "massage parlors" that it was difficult for her to find legitimate customers. She answered my questions about the whole process. She explained what to wear, and how the draping worked. It became clear that I had nothing at all to fear and I made an appointment to try a massage the following week.

I was of course quite nervous when I went for that first massage, but within a few minutes, I felt all of that tension melt away. There is just no way you can feel anxious while a trained massage therapist works on your body. You can feel the stress being pushed out of your muscles.

As I started making regular appointments and my body became more receptive to massage, I began to feel a new sensation. When certain areas of my body were massaged, I would experience different emotions. Particularly my stomach seemed to contain many locked up feelings. As Beth worked my stomach muscles, I would feel a wave of sadness wash over me. It was if I had "stored" emotions in my body rather than letting go of them.

It seemed particularly interesting that the feelings seemed to be stored in my stomach. Could stuffing myself with food be an attempt to massage my stomach from the inside out?

I thought about all of the feelings that I have in my stomach. That is the place were I would always feel sadness or fear. Whenever I had one of those "sinking feelings", it was in my stomach. I'd never made the connection that maybe I was eating to get rid of those unpleasant feelings, at least not physically.

Massage seemed to release things that had been stored in me for years. I never knew why exactly, but it was not unusual to find tears in my eyes after a massage. It wasn't that it was unpleasant and as I became better friends with Beth I wasn't embarrassed. I didn't try to analyze or hide those feelings, just experience them. After a massage, I would feel physically lighter as if all of those feelings that had been weighing me down were gone. The sessions really were quite therapeutic.

Over the years, I met other massage therapists and have tried to keep it a regular part of my life, but I've never quite gotten over the irony of being stuck on a jury and then having something quite wonderful come out of what initially appeared to be a burden. Having a week to "interview" a massage therapist gave me the resources to take the next step in my pursuit of stress reduction.

This illustrates another point worth making: by being clear about your intentions, the ways and means will follow, even if they are not obvious at first. Chance favors the prepared mind. If you know what you truly want, when the time comes you will be able to get it. I doubt that I would have gotten to know Beth at all if I hadn't been clear about my desire to get a massage. I probably would have just gone on with the trial and moved on in life. However, I was clear about what I wanted, and even though I couldn't find a solution to obtain my goal initially, a solution eventually presented itself. Once I knew what I wanted, I was able to follow the path once it appeared.

It is not always necessary to see the path that accommodates your intentions. Just be aware of your intentions and the rest will fall into place when the time comes.

Yoga

Massage was great and meditation intriguing, but I wanted to learn about yoga as well. Variety is everything when it comes to stress reduction. So, once again I visited the bookstore. There are many books on yoga. It is another area, like meditation, that can be approached either spiritually or clinically. That creates a bit of confusion sometimes for people that don't really understand what yoga is about. I have heard of churches sometimes banning yoga classes from their premises in fear of letting strange eastern religions into the minds of their congregation.

To add to the confusion, there are different types of yoga, but the version that we are interested in is called Hatha Yoga. It deals strictly with stretching and relaxation, in balanced and controlled motions. This is accomplished through a routine of physical poses (asanas) which have been developed over many, many years to stretch different parts of the body creatively.

The books that I bought were marginally more useful than the massage books. At least this was something that I could do by myself. The book that I've grown to like the most was *The Runner's Yoga Book* by Jean Couch. It is designed to provide poses that are useful to runners in their stretching programs, but it is not much different from any other yoga program, and would be useful to anybody interested in yoga, not just runners.

The stretches are sorted by the region of the body that they affect, making it easy to pick and choose a personalized routine. What makes this book especially useful is that it is full of excellent photographs showing each step of a stretch. It is also bound so that it can be laid open on the floor while the reader does the pose. That was a big improvement over the paperbacks that I first tried reading. It was maddening to get half-way into a pose and then have the little paper back flop shut, leaving me stranded. *The Runner's Yoga Book* is extremely well thought out and organized.

Nevertheless, even with a good book, yoga just didn't seem to meet my expectations. It really isn't a self-study kind of discipline. I realized that I would be better off to try taking a course.

I had no idea what "yoga people" would be like. Images of that old TV show Kung Fu came to mind. I had visions of a yogi calling me "grasshopper" and quoting Confucius. Once again, that wasn't how it turned out.

I picked a class that turned out to be delightful. The woman teaching it was quite inspiring. She had just the right mix of the traditional yoga philosophy and the modern reality. She could turn herself into a pretzel, but always paced the class appropriately and made each student feel that they were doing well, no matter how much success they would have with a particular stretch. Just like with a massage, my fears of looking foolish or not knowing what to do vanished in the hands of a pro.

As much as Ruby, the instructor, stressed that we shouldn't compare our progress to others, only to ourselves, I couldn't help being impressed by her grace and flexibility. It was only after I had known her for a while that I found out that she was well into her 70s and also taught a course in belly dancing. Talk about a paradigm shift! I would have never guessed her age to be in that range; she looked and acted much younger. It would appear that all of the wondrous benefits of yoga are not at all overstated. (No, I never took her Belly Dancing course—at least not yet.)

In taking a course, I found myself working much harder on the yoga stretches. I didn't give up quite as easily and I took the time to feel the stretch and focus on my body. After an hour of yoga, I could barely remember anything that was bothering me before the class. And when I did think of something, I was able to view it in a new, more rational light.

I also experienced the same emotional release that I felt with massage. Again, stretches that involved my abdomen always released a rush of feelings that I was unaware of before. Where massage was a passive activity, yoga was active. Yoga is almost like having an "internal" massage. It can work on areas of the body that a massage leaves untouched. I would leave the class feeling lighter, and taller! It was not unusual to have to re-adjust my rearview mirror in the car on the drive home: more evidence of the toll that stress takes on our bodies. It is no wonder that Ruby seemed so spry!

Dance

Dance is considered another form of stress reduction. Rhythmic movements of the body coordinated with music produce a stress reducing effect. I have never tried dance, at least not so far. I did get as far as watching a dance group, but my inhibitions kept me on the sidelines. A friend of mine who is interested in Contra Dancing (a variation of Square Dancing) took me to see what it was about. They offered a free lesson for any newcomers, but I was still way too shy. There are many dance groups focusing on different styles from Square dancing to Cajun, and most offer free lessons for anybody interested. Someday...

Tai Chi

I also want to mention tai chi. I have never tried this, but people that I have met learning about the Cornerstones recommend it. It is sort of a "low impact" form of yoga, mixed with rhythmic movements put together into routines. It is typically done outside. I visited San Francisco once and was surprised to see a huge gathering in a park of people doing Tai Chi. There were hundreds, all moving silently and in sync with each other. It was relaxing just to watch. It is something that I will probably pursue someday in my never-ending search for stress reduction.

The Reattachment of the Body

I want to mention the relationship of massage, yoga, dance, and tai chi to the connection of the mind and the body. I think that they are especially useful to a fat person, because most of us have disconnected our minds from our bodies.

Fat people will spend much time and money on their hair and makeup, as well as developing their personalities, but feel like a disembodied spirit when it comes to the rest of their physical selves. We tend to run from mirrors and cameras or anything else that reminds us that we even have bodies.

I would walk around mirrors in department stores rather than past them. If I couldn't avoid them, I would look in another direction. I can even remember instinctively cringing when I watched a television show where a character would walk past a mirror. At some irrational level, I feared that the mirror on the TV screen might also catch my reflection and give me an unwanted glimpse of myself lying on the couch. As impossible as that would be to actually happen, my instincts still flinched, making me aware of my self-loathing.

I was not truly aware of the disconnection until I began to experiment with some of the more physical forms of stress reduction. I never really was aware of my denial of my body until I had to do something that required me to make use of it, especially in public. It was quite uncomfortable, but very healthy too. It helped me reconnect my brain to the rest of me, and to get my whole self functioning in harmony.

The more I put myself "out there", the more I realized that it really didn't matter too much. The more I took on new activities, the more I felt "part" of the world and less ashamed of myself. Certainly as I lost weight this became less threatening, but the old behaviors were still there. It takes a long time to reconnect, and the more activities that promote that, the better.

However, at all times, it is very important to be aware of where you are in the process. Like I said, to this day I'm uncomfortable with the idea of dancing in public. Looking foolish or doing the wrong thing still haunts me. Someday I think it will be within the realm of possibility, and it will give me an entirely new area to explore, but not yet.

Other Stress Reduction Options

I mentioned saunas, whirlpools, and hot baths as another possibility. Simply locking myself in the bathroom in a hot tub of water can be one of the simplest and easiest forms of stress reduction. As un-masculine as it may be, I have invested in a supply of different bubble bath soaps and like to get the water as hot as I can stand it, and just float away. Saunas and whirlpools produce a similar effect, if you have access to them.

Also, never overlook the value of long, quiet stroll through your neighborhood in the early morning or evening as a great way to unwind. Some people taking the Cornerstone class have even managed to talk their spouses into accompanying them and it has turned into a pleasant daily ritual.

But, as I said at first, just giving yourself 10 minutes to lie down and take some deep breaths or visualize can be extremely powerful, even if it doesn't seem like it at the time.

Living in the Moment Exercise

One of the most interesting things that you can do to get yourself re-aligned when stressed-out is to spend a day (or better yet an entire weekend) living from moment to moment. This can take some planning to work out, but it is tremendously energizing if you can manage it.

The idea is to set aside some time with absolutely no plans, no commitments, no intentions, nothing. It doesn't matter how much of a backlog of chores you have, or how many appealing offers you might get beforehand, you must isolate yourself from any sort of commitments or planning. You then spend the day living from moment to moment, doing only what appeals to you at that particular instant.

Turn off your alarm clock. Wake up when you are ready. Forget planned meals. Eat when you are hungry, and then, eat exactly what you are hungry for. If that means going to the store at 2:00 p.m. to buy a particular item that you have developed a craving for, then go get it. If it means going to a restaurant for something, then go. Every moment of the day, ask yourself what it is you are wanting right then and then give it to yourself.

Unplug your telephone and let an answering machine take your calls. If you get in the mood later to check messages, do it—but only if you are genuinely in the mood. If watching television appeals to you, do it. If seeing a movie appeals to you, do it, but don't plan it. Pick up the paper to check the listings only when you are in the mood and then decide what movie appeals to you. Don't plan to see a particular movie in advance, do it only if it seems like a good idea at the time.

Don't plan any of this. Wait until the moment to decide what you want to do. Sit quietly and really tune into yourself to see what you are truly wanting. Literally live from moment to moment and experience what you are genuinely seeking at that instant.

Ideally, you should do this for an entire weekend. Go to bed only when you are tired, not because it's time. Wake up only when you are rested. If reading a book late into the evening seems like a good idea, then read. If you are hungry, then eat, but only if you are hungry, and then only what you are hungry for whether it makes sense or not.

This is not as simple as it sounds. Even if we live alone, our lives are scheduled, planned, and committed far in advance. We make plans with friends days in advance for things that we want to do, but when the time comes, it might not be all that appealing and therefore not all that satisfying. The point of the exercise is to be totally spontaneous. If visiting a particular friend appeals to you, then call them, but don't plan it. If it doesn't work out, then go on to whatever else feels appealing.

Of course, it is not realistic to live like this, but it is tremendously energizing to do it from time to time. It has the effect of re-aligning our energy with our actions. When I have used this technique, I'm always shocked at what I feel like doing. Some things are predictable. A movie that I've wanted to see seems appealing and I check the paper and head off to the next showing. Other days I'll spend just reading and reading, late into the evening.

Oddly, it is not unusual for me to feel like doing some chore that I've been putting off. After a few hours of living in the moment, vacuuming the floor might jump into my mind as something that I want to do. Cleaning the garage, for example, has appealed to me. This only happens after I've truly accepted that I'm free to do exactly what I want, and not when I feel some sort of guilt or frustration about not doing the chore. It is amazing what we find ourselves wanting, when we give ourselves the chance.

If you don't live alone, this probably seems completely impossible, but you are someone who would probably benefit the most from this exercise. When I first heard about this concept, I was still married. It took some doing, but it resulted in one of the most insightful and relaxing weekends I've ever had. My wife and children took some time and went to visit family. I just floated from moment to moment for a weekend. It was incredible. I did the most mundane things and enjoyed them thoroughly. I worked in the yard. I took clothes to the dry cleaner. I saw several movies, read books I'd been ignoring, ate very strange things, and I felt like a million dollars.

Giving ourselves permission to be ourselves, if only for a day, is incredibly difficult and incredibly rewarding. It goes completely against our modern century culture and really takes effort to push back all of the "shoulds" and "shouldn'ts", but it is well worth it. The rush of energy lasts for days afterwards, even after we climb back into our stressed-out, over-committed lives.

Pursue the Adventure!

Make your pursuit of stress reduction an adventure. Stress isn't something that you find a simple solution to and that is the end of it. Sometimes a technique that has been working fine will start to get boring or won't produce the effect that you need. Then it is time switch.

Take time to get to know the people you meet along the path to stress reduction. They probably will live in an entirely different paradigm from yours. You can learn things about yourself by looking at things from a different perspective. You can adopt new ideas into your own paradigm that you would have never thought of before.

Stress reduction really is quite enjoyable, but I suspect you will experience what I have—the more that you need it, the more excuses your body will find to resist it. Be prepared for this and take notice if it begins to happen.

Rely on your journal to track whatever stress reduction activity you use on a particular day and compare your resistance to it with what is happening in your life. If you see that many days have passed and you have done little to reduce stress, view that as a leading indicator of real trouble. A serious binge is probably just around the corner. Get to work immediately. Figure out what is happening and focus your journal writing on the subject. Do something!

Suggestions

- When you come home in the evening, lie down for 10 minutes and picture yourself as you are becoming. This is a good time to focus on your new paradigm.

- Try out different kinds of relaxing music or guided meditation recordings.

- Periodically, spend a day (or two) with absolutely no plans. Do only what pops into your mind at that moment.

- Take a yoga class.

- Get a massage.

- Try a dance group (such as Contra or Square dancing) that offers free lessons.

- Try meditation.

- If you have young children, make a game out of your quiet time. Include them in your 10 minutes of silence, or hang a "do not disturb" sign on your bedroom door.

- Realize that if you feel tired, you probably are just stressed-out and will have new energy after using a stress reduction technique.

- Watch your journal for leading indicators of stress overload—particularly what you've been eating.

- Take short little breaks when you feel frustrated.

- Realize that the more you feel like you don't want to reduce stress, the more you need to.

- Acquire a taste for adventure!

Favorite Excuses

- I don't have the time.
- I don't have any stress in my life.
- I'm not willing to let anyone touch me or see me during a massage.
- Yoga/meditation is satanic.
- I'm too tense to relax.
- I'm too tired when I get home.
- I relax when I watch television at night.
- I'm naturally a high-strung person.
- I'll just fall asleep using a stress reduction technique

Add your favorite excuses here!

- _____
- _____
- _____
- _____
- _____
- _____
- _____
- _____
- _____
- _____
- _____
- _____
- _____

6

Cornerstone III: Fitness

The Concrete Cornerstone

If Stress Reduction is the most abstract Cornerstone, then Fitness could be considered the most concrete. It is quantifiable, measurable, and it will completely shatter your old, self-defeating fat paradigm if you'll let it.

Nothing contradicts the image of a fat person more than someone taking specific action to improve his or her fitness. Nothing will confront your old ideas and belief system more than *letting* yourself be physically fit.

Fitness is quite tangible and within a very short period of time will produce amazing results, if you approach it properly. For that matter, it will produce amazing results if you approach it at all.

If you are reading this paragraph, you are way ahead of the game. Many, many fat people will have already skipped ahead in the book having decided that they can't be physically fit, while anxiously rushing through to find the "secret formula" of weight loss. But if you can stick with me for a while, you might be surprised what you can accomplish and find a whole new person lurking inside you that you never even dreamt could exist in your body.

Believe It or Not

Believe it or not, you already are physically fit. Everybody is at some level of fitness or they would already be dead, and I'm assuming that you are not reading this book posthumously. The question is what level of fitness you want to be, not whether or not you are fit.

Most of us merely accept our level of fitness, and accept its decline as time goes by. We assume that as we get older we will be less fit and that our health will slowly decay. Certainly, nobody will live forever and our bodies do in fact wear out, but not in the way we think, or at least not as passively as we think.

When I ran in the New York City Marathon, there were two people well into their 80's running the course. There were also people running with physical handicaps such as artificial legs or with crutches. There were even people without legs who rolled wheel chairs along for 26.2 miles.

Even after years of running, I wasn't prepared for the eclectic assortment of people I met running that marathon. I had always thought that marathoning was for a select group of super athletes. As I was training for the race, I wasn't sure that I really belonged in such an event. I was wrong. There are no limits if you want something. None.

Without realizing it, we tend to view fitness as something in the future. It is a line that is off in the distance, waiting to be crossed, and one that we will probably never cross. We'd all like to be "physically fit", but have no interest in the physical "torture" that we have to endure to "get there".

But the paradigm shift that you must make with the Fitness Cornerstone is to accept the reality that you already are fit to some degree. The question is to what degree? Where do you want to be and what are you willing to do to get there?

You may have thought that you simply want to weigh less, but we've already discussed what it is that you truly want. Hopefully you've realized that you probably want to look and feel better physically, so that you can move into a life that will be more satisfying.

Becoming *more fit* is a big part of the equation. It is *movement* along the fitness path that you seek, not some distant point down the road that you must reach. When you start moving your level of fitness, things begin to happen quickly. Your self-esteem skyrockets, you sleep better, your appetite changes, you have more energy, and your overall sense of well-being becomes much, much better.

And, all of these good things happen almost right away. They aren't things that happen when you "become fit". They are things that happen when you move your level of fitness even slightly in a positive direction.

The Fat Kid Nobody Wanted on the Team

I grew up in Wisconsin during the 1960s. Those were the days of the Vince Lombardi Green Bay Packers reign over the world of professional football. It seemed that was all we heard about. People planned their lives around the big games. Nobody would plan any event that might conflict with a Packer game. Funerals, weddings, and baptisms all had to be scheduled around the games, at least if you wanted to have anyone show up. Even some of the churches offered what was jokingly called a "football mass". This was a brief 20-minute service that allowed you to sleep late, go to mass, and then get back home in time for the pre-game show. Even God, it seemed, knew what was most important—worshipping athletic ability.

Every little boy was expected to want to play sports, to dream about growing up to be a football star. Every teacher in school seemed to lecture about how wonderful football was. My hometown had a super high school team that annually seemed to win the state championship. We should be so proud!

But the problem was that I had absolutely no coordination for any sport and therefore almost no interest in playing. I was fat (or husky as they liked to call it to make it sound better). I couldn't run fast. I couldn't throw or catch a ball very well. Yet I, like everyone else, was held to the same standards. I was subjected to the humiliation of not being chosen until last during gym class when choosing teams. I was required to play sports by teachers and parents who, with my best interest at heart, claimed that sports should be such an important component in my self-worth.

There was no way to hide it; nobody wanted me on their team. It didn't matter which sport. I was fat. Sports were to mean everything for a boy and therefore I was nothing.

I died a thousand deaths each day in gym class. I was always one of the ones that nobody wanted. To make matters worse, frequently the team that I wound up on would be designated "skins" which meant I had to play without my T-shirt exposing my body for all to see. And on the very worst days, the girl's gym class would be meeting right next to us. I wanted to die of shame.

Softball was just as awful. When I'd come to the plate, everybody would "move in" with a nasty grin. It didn't really matter; I couldn't hit the ball anyway. And, if by some miracle I did manage to tap it, I couldn't waddle fast enough to first base. If I were in the outfield, I couldn't catch the ball or throw it once I chased it down.

I can remember working out a deal with the team leader (the one stuck with me) when we played softball. In the batting rotation, I would just never move up. I would sort of stay at the end of the line and let the previous batter get in front of me. If the other team wasn't watching, we could go the whole game without them noticing. But, if they did, I would be forced to bat and another round of humiliation would ensue.

The athletes got all of the praise and the perks of high school—the letter jackets, the trophies, their pictures in the newspaper. They were everything and I was nothing.

This became the basis of my education about fitness. If it was athletic, it was competitive and full of humiliation. How many calories does humiliation burn?

The Athlete

To me, an athlete was someone whose knuckles dragged on the ground, who had a sloping forehead, and who pronounced the word "football" without a "t": foo-ball. An athlete was a person who quoted Vince Lambardi ad nauseam. "Winning isn't everything, it's the only thing!", "Nice guys finish last!", "If winning weren't important, they wouldn't keep score!", on and on.

Athletics was about competition and beating someone else. It was about pain, both physical and emotional, and it wasn't about me. It was a talent that I didn't have. I didn't need any more humiliation; I already had plenty.

To me, an athlete was something I wasn't and would never be. It was for other people—healthy people—not for fat people.

Fitness in a Nutshell

It was well over 10 years since my final high school gym class when I first learned about the Fitness Cornerstone. The instructions were simple. Anything that got your heart pumping and made you sweat for 20 minutes, three times a week, would qualify.

What a concept! There was nothing about beating somebody, nothing about winning. Just elevate the heart rate for a little while and that was it. I could manage that, I thought. I could easily sweat for 20 minutes 3 times a week. It wasn't something I particularly wanted to do, but I knew that if I wanted my ultimate goal, it was worth a try. My paradigm had shifted and I was ready to try something different.

First Attempt

As easy as the Fitness Cornerstone sounded, I soon realized that it wasn't going to be so simple. I initially decided that I would try jogging as my form of fitness. I'm not sure what it was about running that appealed to me, but I decided that that was what I was going to try. I cut off some old blue jeans, put on a big baggy T-shirt and some old tennis shoes and headed out the door.

Now, you have to picture this: I weighed close to 300 pounds, my legs couldn't really support anything much past a slow, pounding trot and my heart and lungs were in worse shape. I will never forget that first attempt at running. I could not make it more than half of a block before I gave up. The attempt was more like a near-death experience than a workout. The pain was incredible. Everything seemed to get dim. I was wheezing. My heart was pounding so loudly I thought that it would come through my chest. I'd never attempted anything quite like that in my life before and I was never further away from being able to run than I was at that moment.

I had the pain part down. Now for the humiliation. I didn't have to look far. As I lumbered down the street, people couldn't help noticing. This wasn't the typical jogger that you barely notice running along the side of the street, this was more like something from the movie *Jurassic Park*. Somebody must have cloned a strange, large beast and turned it loose on the streets. It certainly didn't belong there. Apparently, nobody had ever seen anything like this before. People felt obliged to roll down their car windows and yell things at me—things that are too painful to recount even now. Children playing in their yards stopped and taunted me with insults. It was hell.

What I know now, but didn't then, is that I was disturbing their universe. I was challenging their paradigm and they didn't like it. Fat people don't try to be fit. They're fat. They go on diets and then go off diets. They stay home except to go out for ice cream and groceries. So here was something that just shouldn't be and they felt they had an obligation to put things right again. As mean as they were, it was all quite understandable. Get this guy off the street and we can have the world back the way it should be! They were performing a public service.

As much hell as running was, I wasn't going to give up. I was determined to do this three times a week. But which times? I wasn't very good with agreements at first. I didn't realize that I was probably going to thwart my own intentions, to avoid both emotional and physical pain. I quickly found my agreements crumbling.

Monday:
  Well, this can wait for a better day, Mondays are hell anyway.

Tuesday:
  Still plenty of time to get three runs in this week, maybe tomorrow.

Wednesday
  Nothing

Thursday
  Nothing

Friday:
  Whoops. I guess I have to go today, Saturday and Sunday if I'm going to keep my agreement. But wait a minute! Who says a week has to start on Monday? Maybe I should be on a fiscal week and start my weeks on Wednesday. Yeah, that's it! I'll just start this next Wednesday...

As you might expect, my running died quickly. It probably was a good thing, now that I think about it. Back in those days I was in no shape to attempt something like that anyway. As sincere as my intentions were, they just weren't realistic. My agreements were bound to fail.

Disaster Recovery

By the time that I realized that I was lying to myself about my fitness agreements, I was already far enough into the other Cornerstones that I wasn't ready to just give up on fitness. It was the first time that I experienced how the Cornerstones can support each other. Even though I wasn't running, I was keeping up with my journal and I was being honest with myself about my progress. I was spending 10 minutes a day relaxing and visualizing just where I was and where I was going. I wasn't going to give up.

I took a hard look at myself and decided what I could realistically accomplish at that point in time. I realized that being physically fit wasn't some distant event in the future. It didn't matter where I was or how bad off I was; it only mattered that I start moving in a healthier direction.

I decided that public humiliation wasn't really a necessity for fitness. I needed something private. Also, I needed something less demanding that running. Running was way beyond my abilities and maybe always would be, I thought. But it didn't matter. I just needed to get my heart pumping three times a week. That was all.

After much thought, I decided to buy an exercise bicycle. It seemed plausible that I might be able to work out, if I could do it without anybody knowing. I didn't know anything about the bikes and spent a long time comparing prices and features. Even looking at exercise equipment in a store made me feel a little silly, as if I didn't belong there at all. But some of the bikes had great big seats, big enough for my great big butt, and I thought that the manufacturer must have had a fat person in mind when they designed that particular model. Maybe it was okay for me to be shopping there after all.

I finally bought the cheapest model I could find. It had almost no features, just a timer and an odometer/speedometer. I really wasn't ready to invest a lot of money in this. I wasn't sure how long I would be riding it; I was only willing to try.

I told nobody (except my wife) what I was doing, no friends or co-workers. I set the bike up in the middle of the room, closed the doors to the room, and asked my wife to leave me alone during my workouts. I even pulled the drapes on the windows shut, so that nobody could see me from the street. This was going to be a private event. If I failed, it would be my failure, not a failure because of somebody else humiliating me.

The exercise bike had another "plus" in addition to its ability to be kept a secret. The difficulty could be adjusted to an appropriate level for the rider. The workout could be as strenuous or as moderate as desired. It didn't matter how out of shape or fat I was; I could set the bike to be "just right". Running, by contrast, was always going to be too strenuous for me at that time. I was so huge that the amount of work to move my body down the street was way beyond my level of fitness, but the bike could challenge me in just the right way.

I learned that the goal of the workout was to elevate my pulse into what is called the *target zone*. There was a simple calculation (described later) that would yield the proper level of workout for me, and me alone. The target zone concept automatically adjusted to my age and level of fitness. The more out of shape I was, the less work I had to do to elevate my pulse to get the desired effect. There was no risk in overdoing it.

I set the resistance on the bike to just enough so that my heart rate would be above the minimum rate, but below the maximum. It didn't take much in the beginning to achieve that heart rate. The more out of shape I was, the easier it was to get my heart pumping faster. I could set the timer for 20 minutes and check my pulse to make sure I was pedaling hard enough and that was all there was to it.

The nice part about the bicycle was that there was no pounding on my knees as there would be with running. All of that weight was supported by the seat and I could focus my energy on exercising my heart, not ruining my body.

I also found that by turning the stereo on with some of my favorite music, it would really make the workout more appealing. The time would go by much more quickly and the pain didn't seem as great.

Years later, I learned that music is actually a very powerful addition to a workout because it stimulates the right side of the brain. When I was training for the marathon, the training coach explained that the left side of the brain is analytical and the right side creative. When we are running (or whatever), the excuses and discouraging thoughts will all be coming from the left side. By stimulating the right side of the brain by listening to music, humor, or using a visualization technique, the flow of self-defeating thoughts will diminish and the feeling of pain will be reduced, if not eliminated.

Still, I had the problem of determining which three days I was going to do my workouts. By using my journal, I realized that when I tried to work out in the evenings I tended to find excuses and not keep my agreements. By the time I was finished with a day of work, I was stressed-out enough that I had no desire to exercise. Too many other options would have appeared by the time I returned home in the evening for me realistically to expect to keep a fitness agreement.

Mornings, on the other hand seemed to work much better. Not that it was easy. It required getting up an hour earlier than I was used to. But again, by writing in my journal I realized that no matter when I got up in the morning, I still felt tired, so why not get up an hour earlier and get something done as well as feel tired?

In the morning, there were fewer excuses. Once I thought about it, I realized that everything I did from the moment that the alarm clock went off to the moment I sat down at my desk at work was all habit. I rolled out of bed, ate some breakfast, brushed my teeth, shaved, took a shower, got dressed, got in the car, drove the same route, parked in the same spot and went to work. Mornings were simply a string of habits that I had never thought much about before. Why not just add an additional habit?

It worked beautifully. The morning workout became as routine as shaving. I didn't debate whether or not I was going to shave that day, and I didn't debate whether or not I was going to ride my bike. Once it became part of the routine, there was no point in thinking about it anymore.

In fact, I found that I was much better off if I just rode the bike *every* morning. Why not? Three days was the minimum, but why not do more? It actually was easier to do that. It eliminated all the decision-making and quickly became a routine, not a *special* event.

In addition, I found that with a morning workout, I started the day with something for *myself*. I began each 24 hours with something that I had decided was important for me. Nobody else had anything to do with it. It was all mine.

By exercising early in the morning, there was less chance for some external source in my life to mess up my plans. Before anything could go wrong in the day, something had gone right. Before the traffic could get congested, before problems could arise at work, before any sort of unforeseen trouble could get hold of me, I had already claimed the day as mine. The day always began on a positive note. I found that the difference in my outlook for the rest of the day would be radically shifted. No matter how frustrating the day might become, at the core of the day was a positive event and I dealt with problems much more objectively. I was in control of my life; it was no longer in control of me.

The morning workout served as a stimulant. It woke me up and prepared me for what was coming. After about three weeks, my body didn't resist the idea of exercise. It actually started to crave it. I later learned that what was happening was that I was beginning to produce endorphins, a natural pain-killer that is released during exercise. Endorphins also elevate mood. Without knowing it, I was giving myself a shot of "good feelings" that lasted throughout the day. My new behavior was becoming addictive and I was finding myself turning to it, much as I had previously turned to food to find solace.

Competition Re-defined: To Hell with Vince Lombardi!

The exercise bike gave me some other insights into fitness and life in general. I could compete with myself rather than with someone else or someone else's ideas. I began to play games with my workouts. After I became comfortable with a level of fitness, I would begin to push myself just a little harder. I would see if I could manage to pedal just a little further during the same amount of time. I would check my pulse to make sure I was still within the target range, always being careful not exceed it, but working just a little harder. My body started becoming more fit and I was able continually to accomplish more.

On other days, particularly on weekends when I'd have more time, I'd see if I could work out longer—maybe 10 additional minutes. I would do this just out of curiosity, not out of some sense of needing more. I began to tune into myself and my own level of fitness, and then challenge that. I forgot any old Vince Lombardi notions of competition. My competitive drive turned inward. It didn't matter what anybody else could do. This was about me. It wasn't about winning, it was about growth.

The self-competition theme began to creep into all areas of my life. I learned to look at where I was, and who I was, and what I wanted before making any judgments about my abilities. I stopped looking to others to set the rules about what I should be doing. I realized that growth should be the emphasis, not a specific accomplishment. Beating someone else means nothing. Improving yourself means everything. My growth from a couch potato to a marathoner was a huge improvement, and I did it without any comparison to anyone else. It didn't matter how fast or how far anyone else could run. It only mattered what I could do. Period.

Running Revisited

About 18 months into my exercise biking, my cheap bicycle broke. I'll never forget that day. I was pedaling along as usual, but a terrible squealing sound started to come from the wheel. Then, blue oily smoke started to fill the room as the bearings finally gave out and the bike ground to a halt.

The odometer showed over 3000 miles. My $75 bike had been used up. It wasn't really built for that level of usage. Since then, I've made a habit of checking the odometer on any exercise bike I see in someone's home. I have yet to find one with over 200 miles on it and most have less than 100. Apparently, the normal pattern is to buy a bike, ride it a few times, and then quit. The manufacturers must be aware of this and realize there is no need to put much in the way of heavy-duty engineering into their bikes, since nobody is really going to use them anyway. There was no way my bike could take the punishment that I'd been giving it. My bike was dead. I gave it a nice funeral and sat down to think about what to do next.

By this time, I'd lost a lot of weight and my heart and lungs were in significantly better shape. I decided it might be time to give running another shot.

What a difference! I tried running once again and could make it well past the corner where I used to have to stop. Nobody yelled anything at me. My life didn't flash before my eyes. I was a different person. I could put on my running shoes and just go without shame.

I continued to use my pulse rate as a gauge to set my running pace. If it wasn't high enough, I'd speed up. If it got too high, I'd slow down. I would just continue to keep it in the target zone for a 30-minute run and then see how far I would get.

As I got healthier, I could run further in the same amount of time. Before too long, I was able routinely to run about three miles in my 30-minute workout. I'd strap on a portable music player and "zone out" while I ran. And it felt *so* good!

I learned to love to sweat. That probably sounds strange, since most people think of perspiring as something that it is best avoided, but I really got to enjoy it. I felt like I was cleansing myself from the inside out. At the end of a good run, I felt as if I had wrung all of the toxins out of my body, just as if I'd twisted a saturated sponge over the sink.

Further Paradigm Shifts

Even though I ran every day, I still thought of running as something that "other people" did. I had learned to like the privacy of my workouts and never had considered running in a public event.

I was quite shocked when some co-workers invited me to run with them in an upcoming race. Every year in Atlanta, the Peachtree Roadrace is a huge race that is run on the 4th of July. Many, many thousands of people sign-up to run 6.2 miles down Peachtree Road in the heat of July, in front of thousands of onlookers and well-wishers. I'd never considered such a ridiculous thing before and couldn't imagine anyone inviting me to run in it.

I didn't realize that by this time I was beginning to look much more athletic than I ever had in my life. I'd switched jobs and people who hadn't known me before had no idea about my past. They only saw the "new" me, and to them I was a logical choice for the race. I was flattered and terrified. Didn't these people know who I was—a fat out of shape guy that nobody should want on their team? Of course, they didn't know who I was. But then I realized, maybe they *did* know who I was. Maybe I was the one who didn't know who I was anymore.

I'm not sure just what I was thinking, but I agreed at least to try a practice run with them before I committed. I was terrified. I'd never run past 3 miles before and we were going to run 4 to begin. And these were "athletes"—I was going to look like a fool in front of them. What in the world was I thinking?

Somehow, I got up the courage and went along on the practice run. I expected to be left behind, but I found that I could keep up pretty well. I wasn't as fast as they were, but at least I survived with some dignity. And of course this wasn't really about winning. This wasn't the kind of a thing you did to win. In those days there were 25,000 people running the race (it has since grown to 60,000). It was an event, not a race. It didn't matter how fast you were, it just mattered that you did it. I agreed to enter the race and proceeded to begin to worry endlessly about it for the next few months.

I had visions of finishing the course in an ambulance, or at least hours behind the other 24,999 runners. I trained and trained, just to be safe. Before long, I could easily make the 6.2 miles and started to relax a little bit about things.

On the day of the race, all of the old fears came back. This was a big media event. The local TV stations had cameras and helicopters flying overhead. The streets were lined with people. I was scared to death. This made playing softball in front of the girl's gym class seem like nothing.

I remember standing in the crowd, waiting for the race to begin. The excitement was awesome. 25,000 people were waiting to run, many of them for their first time. I knew that I was going to make it. In a sense, I already had made it. I deserved to be there. I'd earned it. I was as much a part of the event as any of those other runners, including the elite "invited" world-class runners who were lined up at the front of the pack.

It took me almost an hour to run that race, but it was one of the most wonderful moments in my life. It was all I could do to keep from crying when I crossed the finish line and picked up my T-shirt. The fat kid had done it.

For months afterwards, I felt so proud. I'd get out a map of the city and just look at the course and at how far I'd run: 6.2 miles! I never in my wildest dreams would have thought that I could have done that. Two years before I was a hopeless fat blob, and now I'd accomplished something that I'd never even considered.

Now What?

Ironically, since I had now moved into such uncharted territory, I brought very few pre-conceived ideas about my limits. Once I had broken through the initial barrier, there seemed as if there were *no* limits.

I went on to participate in many more races and my running time improved. I certainly never even got close to winning, but I never really cared either, it just was a thrill to run. The T-shirts awarded at the end of each race piled up, reminding me of what I was doing.

I started thinking about running even longer distances than 6.2 miles. After a few years, I'd worked myself up to a half-marathon (13.1 miles) and doubled the distance of that first race that I'd run. My paradigm had shifted further. 6.2 miles was nothing, 13.1 miles was something now! Eventually, after a few more years, I began to think the unthinkable—a full 26.2 mile marathon.

Nine years after I'd started the Fitness Cornerstone, history repeated itself and several friends began talking to me about training for the New York City Marathon. I couldn't quite imagine that at first, but then I realized that was always the case. This time, deep down inside, I knew that I could do it, even before I started the training program.

I enrolled in a 6-month training class taught by Olympic runner Jeff Galloway. Even though Jeff is quite a well-known runner with best selling books on the subject, the class wasn't full of super athletes, just everyday people who wanted to accomplish something. We learned all sorts of techniques to keep things interesting and to endure the inevitable pain. For the first time, my daily running routine had to be changed. Jeff stressed the importance of rest days. There was no way my body could take that amount of mileage without time to recover. However, by then I was so thoroughly addicted to running, that I actually had to make agreements *not to run* on certain days; it was as difficult as it had been to agree to run in the beginning when I first waddled out of the door 9 years before.

Everything fell into place. I was lucky to have my name chosen in the lottery to be among the 25,000 people that would be allowed to run the marathon. I flew to New York City for a long weekend and when race day came, I had another one of the most thrilling moments in my life.

The race was broadcast on national television. The grand prize was $50,000. The best athletes from all over the world came to compete, and I would be running with them!

The crowds that line the street to watch the race are breath taking. The noise as you enter Manhattan along First Avenue is deafening. I think what impressed me most was the incredible variety of people in the race. There were people with artificial limbs, people on crutches, people in wheelchairs, even blind people running the distance. Some would take close to 24 hours to finish. Everybody there had a certain spark of achievement in their eyes and I really felt like I belonged.

Crossing the finish line in Central Park was amazing. I'd been running for over 4 hours and was in pain. Still, I had to think about the fact that the fat kid that nobody wanted on the team had just finished the New York City Marathon.

The Funny Thing about Paradigms

Paradigms can cut both ways. When I attended my 20th High School Class Reunion, I hadn't seen anyone from my class in 20 years. Nobody had any idea who I was. I looked completely different. What struck me most of all was that many of the "athletes" that I had once been jealous of, now looked more like I used to. They had become sedentary and had had little luck keeping up their level of fitness. I don't mean to sound smug; it wasn't that I felt that I was better than they were. I still don't put much value in comparison with other people. It was just the power of the paradigm that struck me. They had followed the traditional path, slowing down and switching from participation to observation. The only athletics in their lives were the ones they saw on television. Since I had abandoned my old ways of thinking, without really thinking about it, I had moved into a completely new world. I didn't have a path that was prescribed by somebody else. The only boundaries I knew were the ones that I set myself. All things considered, I think I prefer my approach, even though I never had a date with a cheerleader.

Forget about Calories

People have frequently told me that the way that I must be able to keep my weight off is to burn many extra calories through working out. I don't believe this is true. I average 30 minutes of exercise a day. That is all.

It is common to think that the purpose of exercise is to burn calories. It has been my experience that this is completely untrue. Anybody who has ever looked up the calories burned during 30 minutes of exercise knows that it is hardly worth the bother. All of that work probably wouldn't burn off a decent candy bar, and most overeaters have a lot more than one too many candy bars a day.

After running the marathon, I entered my running time, distance, and my weight into a computer program that calculates how many calories are burned during a workout. In over 4 hours of running 26 miles, I burned only 3500 calories. Any calorie counter knows that 3500 calories equals about 1 pound of fat. So, in all of that work, I managed to burn off only 1 pound! Hypothetically, having been 100 pounds overweight, I would have needed to run 100 marathons to lose the weight that I did according to the computer's calculation.

It is important to realize that the Fitness Cornerstone is not about burning extra calories. There probably is no way you could do enough extra exercise to get rid of any significant amount of fat, at least on a strictly mathematical basis. If you are doing a lot of binge eating, don't look to exercise as a way to undo your indulgence. That isn't how it works.

Set Points

The theory that I like better than the calorie burning theory is the concept of set points. The idea behind set points is that our bodies have an internal setting that regulates our body weight. It controls our metabolism and our appetites to keep our weight at the proper setting. Over the long haul, it doesn't matter how much you undereat or overeat, eventually your set point will kick back in and your body weight will return to "normal", much as a thermostat will turn the furnace back on when the room temperature gets too far away from the proper setting.

Exercise on a regular basis lowers the set point to a healthier setting. It takes about three weeks, but during this time, some inner mechanism re-calibrates the set point in order to accommodate this new "habit". Our bodies come to realize that this new activity is for real and that a much leaner physique is appropriate.

It is not true that exercise increases appetite. It regulates appetite. Sometimes that means increasing it and sometimes that means decreasing it. Either way it is rarely predictable. Sometimes I have found my appetite diminished after I've been on a long run and sometimes I've found myself ravenous. It all just depends on the set point.

There have been times when I've been on vacation and have eaten tremendous amounts of food, but I don't seem to add any weight. It is as if my body "knows" that this isn't the normal routine for me and it can just pass these calories on through without bothering to store them as fat. On the other hand, there have been times when I've undereaten for one reason or another, but my weight doesn't decrease. Later on I just find myself eating more to compensate.

Resting Pulse Rate

An excellent measure of your current set point is your resting pulse rate. This is the rate at which your heart beats when you are completely at rest. The ideal time to check your resting pulse is when you first wake up in the morning. You should be able to feel your pulse in your wrist or in your neck. Count the beats for 15 seconds and then multiply by 4 to get the number of beats per minute. The lower the number, the better.

As your heart gets stronger, it has to beat less frequently to move the same volume of blood, and the pulse rate drops. My resting pulse has dropped from over 90 beats per minute when I first started, down to as low as 53 at the peak of my marathon training.

Track your resting pulse every day in your journal. Long before you see a drop in your weight, you will see a drop in your resting pulse rate. This is a sign that things are changing for the better. Your body is learning a new way of living and it is getting healthier.

On the other hand, if you overdo your workouts, you might find your resting pulse spiking upwards. This is your body warning you that you are pushing too hard.

Additionally, increased levels of stress will send the resting pulse higher. It is important to get to know yourself over the long run and to know what your pattern is. If you regularly have a resting pulse of 70 and then it shoots up to close to 80, slow down. Focus on stress reduction more than on working out so hard. When the resting pulse returns to its normal range, increase the level of workout again.

There are no absolutes when it comes to the resting pulse rate. It can vary widely from person to person. As you might expect, there is no value comparing your rate to anyone else's. The only value is comparing your rate against your own history.

Target Pulse Rate

The obvious warning before starting any new physical workout is to be sure of your current level of health and ability. This probably means a chat with your doctor to review your intentions, particularly if you have any history of heart or other health problems. Some very enlightening tests can be performed that will give you a good idea of how to proceed safely. Twice in my years of running, I have seen people die of heart attacks in the middle of a race. Both times, they were people that had heart conditions lurking that they were unaware of and both were people that undertook too strenuous an exercise regime or didn't prepare properly. Certainly, there is risk in anything, even in crossing the street, but there is no point in taking foolish risks. However, don't ignore the risk of staying fat. Obese people die young more often than healthy people do.

To achieve the correct level of training, it is important to calculate your *target zone heart rate.* This is the rate that you want your heart to beat at for 20 minutes—at least 3 times a week. It varies depending on age, and your doctor may want to alter your level from the calculations presented in the next section.

By elevating your heart rate during a workout, your heart is exercised along with the rest of your body. The level at which you want to do this will decrease as you get older.

If you are willing to spend some money, there are all kinds of fancy devices that will monitor your pulse as you work out. They range in price from $20 up to $200. When I ran the first half-marathon, I wore a pulse monitor and used it as sort of a speedometer. It had a setting that would beep when my heart rate dropped below the minimum or rose above the maximum. Rather than worry about how fast I was running, I just made sure I kept my heart pumping at the correct level throughout the race. Ironically, this was one of the races where another runner died of a heart attack. It was one time when I was quite glad that I was being so careful to watch my level of exertion.

Fancy devices are not necessary. All that is required is that you check your pulse about every 10 minutes when working out. Don't check it for more than 10 seconds. After just a few moments, the rate will begin to drop and give you false readings. Simply stop, feel your pulse while looking at a watch, and count the beats for 10 seconds. It is easiest to calculate your Target Zone so that you know what your rate should be for a 10-second count, rather than for an entire minute; the math is just easier. But if you prefer, you can take your 10 second count and multiply it by 6 to yield the actual rate per minute.

Five minutes after a workout, your pulse rate should be below 120 (or 20 for a ten second count), or your workout was too difficult. A good measure of the strength of your heart is how quickly it returns to its resting pulse rate.

The following section details the formula to compute your personal Target Zone and includes an example of the calculation. By using this simple formula, you will have the key to a highly effective workout that will always yield the proper level of exertion for your current level of fitness.

Heart Rate Target Zone Calculation

1. Calculate maximum heart rate:
   220–age

2. Calculate low target zone rate:
   Maximum x 70%

3. Calculate high target zone rate:
   Maximum x 80%

4. Divide the target zones by 6 to get a 10-second pulse count.

Example: Age 35

1. Maximum: 220–35 = 185 (per minute, 31 per 10 seconds)

2. Low Target: 185 x .7 = 130 (per minute, 22 per 10 seconds)

3. High Target: 185 x .8 = 148 (per minute, 25 per 10 seconds)

4. Target range for 10 seconds is 22 to 25 beats

- Keep heart rate in the target zone for at least 20 minutes, 3 times a week.

- Take pulse for only 10 seconds to verify target zone.

- 5 minutes after finishing, pulse should be below 120 (20 for a 10 second count) or the workout was too difficult.

- Track resting pulse immediately after waking in the morning. It should begin to drop gradually as fitness increases.

- Discuss any plans for physical activity with your doctor before beginning a rigorous training program!

The Choice of an Exercise Activity

Any aerobic activity is valid for your choice of an exercise activity. Anything that elevates your pulse rate into the target zone is valid as an exercise routine. It really doesn't matter what it is as long as your pulse rate is increased and sustained for at least 20 minutes.

Ironically, many body builders have poor heart rates because they don't exercise their heart while they lift weights. They have great looking bodies, but are actually in lousy shape unless they also use an aerobic activity to keep their heart and lungs healthy.

You can vary your activity also. You might use jogging, an exercise bike, brisk walking, a stair climbing machine, or anything else that appeals to you and switch back and forth on different days to keep things interesting. I still use an exercise bike when it is raining and I don't feel like getting soaked. I read recently that a study found that treadmills tend to give the most vigorous workouts without the user being aware of it, so if avoiding at least the perception of exertion is important for you, you might want to try one. But whatever activity you choose, just make sure you monitor your heart rate and keep track of your activity in your journal.

On the basis of my experience, I would recommend that you do something every day, just to reinforce the habit. The effects will come more quickly and you will spend less time debating which days are going to be your workout days. Also, I prefer the mornings, as I mentioned before, simply because it gets you off to a good start for the day. But, there is no rule about this, whatever works for you is right. Lunchtime or evenings are just as useful and can be very helpful in relieving the day's stress or releasing pent-up frustration and anger.

Many people use walking as their aerobic activity. This is fine, but just be careful that you are not simply strolling along, kidding yourself that you are working out. Walking is very pleasant, but if you are not huffing and puffing, it should probably be used as a stress reduction technique, not for a workout.

And again, let me suggest the use of music to keep your right brain active and your left brain quiet with its endless supply of reasons to quit. Get a portable music player and get to it!

As far as exercise equipment goes, I wouldn't spend a lot of money at first. I see many people go out and buy the most deluxe model, only to lose interest very quickly. Unless you already have a lot of experience with exercise, you probably don't know what is going to appeal to you over the long haul. Buy something cheap, or better yet borrow equipment from a friend who is "currently out of the habit of working out".

My first bike was quite cheap and didn't last. But it did its job and I've since replaced it with a more industrial strength model that has survived the years. I had no idea when I started how sincerely I was going to be working out. That first bike matched my intentions at that moment.

Exercise classes can be fun too, if you can stand the idea of public exhibition of your efforts. Some health clubs offer classes for the overweight, but be careful about signing long term contracts. There are plenty of people out there who know all about the good intentions of the out-of-shape and are waiting to slim your wallet more than your body. Take it slowly and get to know yourself as you go. New horizons will continue to appear over time.

And lastly, be careful of the exercise buddy. You don't want your intentions tied to someone else who is going to lose interest and mess up your training. This is about *your* life. Comparing yourself with anyone else might serve more to discourage you, or even hold you back from reaching your true potential. If you do use a buddy, have a plan for what you will do if your buddy doesn't uphold their end of the deal.

Further Studies

There are endless books on the subject of aerobic exercise and I encourage you to seek them out to enhance your interest in the subject. Any book by Kenneth Cooper will go into great depth about the physiology of exercise and how to set up a good routine. Just don't become discouraged with a training plan that is too elaborate. Focus on your heart rate and let that be your guide. All you need to know about exercise is presented in the section on the Heart Rate Target Zone Calculation.

Suggestions

- Exercise first thing in the morning. Mornings are pure habit, making new behaviors easier to cultivate.

- Exercise on an empty stomach.

- Exercise everyday initially to build the habit.

- Allow 3 weeks for changes to start to take place.

- Use music while exercising to stimulate the right brain and stem the flow of self-defeating thoughts.

- Take your resting, active, and recovery pulse religiously. Exercise in your range for at least 20 minutes. Track your resting pulse.

- If you are embarrassed, exercise in private, particularly at first.

- Use a machine like an exercise bike, rowing machine, or stair climber. This is particularly helpful while you are overweight.

- Compete with mileage, time, or other external measurements, but not with other people.

- Fantasize while exercising. Think about who you are becoming and who you want to be.

- Any type of activity that elevates your pulse into the target range for 20 minutes is adequate.

- Trying letting anger surface while you are working out, it can supply a lot of energy.

- Think of perspiration as cleansing yourself from the inside out.

- Acquire a taste for adventure!

Favorite Excuses

- I don't have the time.

- I'm not an athlete.

- I'm too old.

- I'm too young.

- I'm too fat.
- I'm too tired.
- I hate exercise.
- I hate to sweat.
- I have too many physical restrictions.
- I run around enough with my children/job as it is.
- People would laugh at me.
- I don't want to feel pain.
- My sex life would suffer.
- I wouldn't have the energy for anything else.

Add your favorite excuses here!

- _____
- _____
- _____
- _____
- _____
- _____
- _____
- _____
- _____
- _____
- _____
- _____

7

Cornerstone IV: Nutrition

What to Eat—The Magic Formula

If you are like most people, you probably have flipped right to this page to find out what you are supposed to be eating on this "diet". In every diet book I ever bought, I would read maybe a page or two and then start skimming to find **THE DIET.** I was so eager to find that magic potion that would solve my problems that I would ignore anything else that the book had to say. I would then mark the particular page that had **THE DIET** so that I could return to it quickly and never pay much attention to the rest of the book.

Well, if that is what you've done with this book, forget it. You can hunt forever but you are not going to find a word about what foods you are *supposed* to eat. There is no current nutritional wisdom here. There is no state-of-the-art information about saturated fats, no political arguments in favor of vegetarianism, no tofu recipes, no grapefruit diets, no low-carb, no high-carb, no low-fat, no zone, just reality.

Getting Real

Reality. Let's face it; that is where we all live, even though most of us hate it and expend tremendous amounts of energy pretending we live somewhere else. But ultimately, there is no denying it. Reality will rear its ugly head whenever we want it to the least. It will color our best intentions and undo our most ingenious plans. Terrifying as it is, reality is everywhere.

And, the reality is, *you already know what to eat.* Face it, *you* already know what *you* are doing that is causing your problem. You just don't want to admit it. You already know everything you need to know about food, *you just don't like what you know.* You are eager to find some fact that you've missed that will change everything without changing anything. Frustrating, isn't it?

How to Quickly Identify Non-Fattening Foods

I have devised a simple little test that I use to determine what I should eat and what I shouldn't. When deciding if I should allow myself to eat something, I think back and try to remember if I've ever seen a thin person eating that particular food. If I have, then it's okay to eat. If I haven't, well this could be that unique food that will cause me to blimp up like a huge balloon and I'd better stay away from it, or at least get a thin person to test it for me first.

So far, I haven't found any foods that I haven't seen thin people eat, so I have pretty much been eating what I want for the last 20+ years. But you never know, lurking around the corner could be that deadly fat food, just waiting for an unsuspecting thin person to take a bite and explode into obesity, spraying buttons and shreds of clothing all around the room.

The Ever Changing Science of Healthy Eating

It seems barely a week goes by that we don't hear about some new study telling us what not to eat, some new information that confuses us further and adds to our feelings of despair. This certainly has gone on my entire life and I don't expect it to stop anytime soon.

I don't doubt the scientific validity of good nutrition, but science has a way of factoring out the reality of life and it doesn't really tell us much that we can use on a regular basis. And the reality is, no matter how poorly the human race has eaten throughout history, there have always been thin people as well as fat people. Back when we thought that we needed meat with every meal, back when we didn't realize that fat and fried foods were unhealthy, back when nobody worried about how much sugar they were getting, there were thin people eating lousy foods and staying thin.

For example, the other day, a new study was released revealing that the tub of movie theater popcorn that I was innocently eating was actually loaded with the same amount of fat as 9 Big Macs! I couldn't believe that. I didn't want to believe that. Popcorn was part of the total entertainment package, how could it be so bad? But there it was to be believed.

Well, maybe movie theater popcorn is bad. The strange thing is that it never made me fat. I've been eating it for years now, long after I lost all of my fat, and it never made me get fat again. I didn't see it make anybody else in the theater getting fat either. We all looked pretty much the same when we left the theater as when we came in.

So what do I do with this new information about the deadly popcorn? Whatever makes sense. I do care about clogging my arteries with fat and maybe that is reason enough to find alternatives, but when it comes to being fat, I can just ignore the whole thing. Whatever else popcorn does to me, I know it won't make me fat. And if you are like most people, that is your primary concern—not being fat.

Don't let yourself become all tangled up in what is good to eat and what isn't. Just when you think you've understood nutrition, the rules will probably change. You know *what* you're doing to make yourself fat, and you know *when* you're doing it. Your goal is to get a handle on your *behavior*, not on your food. There is nothing out there that you can't have. Really.

Eating What You Want

So, you can eat what you want, when you want. But isn't that what you're doing now? Well, not exactly. Chances are you're torturing yourself with guilt and shame. Very possibly, you're on some foolish diet, or at least trying to make yourself eat food you're not particularly interested in. You've probably stocked the refrigerator with carrot sticks that you intend to eat when you want a chocolate bar. How many carrot sticks does it take to equal the satisfaction of a chocolate bar? Is that reality? How do you feel after you eat the carrot stick? Satisfied? How do you feel after you give in and eat the chocolate bar? Guilty? Then what do you do? I'll bet you eat more chocolate, very possibly winding up in a full-blown binge.

Many years ago during my fat years, I was invited to a pizza party with a group of co-workers. It was a special occasion and it was going to be held a popular Italian restaurant that specialized in extremely thick, cheesy, meaty pizzas.

I was caught in a terrible dilemma. I was already several weeks into another attempt at Weight Watchers and I was doing "pretty well". If I had just started the diet, I would have simply stopped, gone to the party, and then restarted the diet. However, I was a good 20 pounds into it and I didn't want to give up and start over. On the other hand, I really wanted to go to that party. These were good friends and I had no reason not to go, and in fact, I very much wanted to go. So, what was I to do?

I brought the problem up with my Weight Watcher's leader. She was very understanding, but didn't give me the special release from the rules of the diet that I'd hoped to obtain. Somehow, I thought that if she said it was okay, that would change things and I would be able to eat what I wanted without undoing any progress on the diet.

She wouldn't give me "permission" to go off the diet for just one night as I'd hoped. She instead talked about just going, having fun, ordering a plain salad instead of pizza, and bringing along my own diet salad dressing for the topping. Oh boy, that sure sounded good. There I would be, just having a great time, watching everyone else eat pizza while I choked down a salad with diet salad dressing. Once again, there would be the Two Category Fat Paradigm—the thin people having fun and the fat guy struggling to fit in.

I thought about just staying home, but that seemed wrong. So, I decided to go ahead and go to the party with my little Tupperware container of "legal" salad dressing. I was as determined as could be, ready for all out war with myself if that is what it took to sit and watch people savoring pizza.

Then, a miracle happened! We got to the restaurant and on the menu, besides the wonderful pizza, listed way down at the bottom was—believe it or not—broiled fish! Good old crappy, broiled fish! What a godsend! I don't know about Weight Watchers today, but back in those days you were supposed to eat 5 Fish Meals a week. I never really did—I hate fish—but you were supposed to eat it. I was lucky to choke down even one Fish Meal a week. But, as if to be rewarded by the diet gods for my good intentions with my salad dressing, I had been given the opportunity to consume yet another Fish Meal rather than simply just there and eat my salad. I could act as if I were at least somewhat "normal"; instead of ordering pizza, I could order broiled fish and not ever haul out my salad dressing container! I could pretend that fish is what I really wanted. Praise the Lord! I could be normal!

I ordered the fish and ignored all of that fantastic pizza. During the whole meal I was planning what I was going to tell my Weight Watcher leader next week about my wonderful dieting experience. I would get to stand up, tell the class about my conquest, and then they would clap and be very impressed with my tremendous dieting abilities. But, deep down inside, I wanted that pizza. The fish just didn't cut it. Every slice of pizza that I saw, I wanted to grab and stuff into my face. I could smell the sauce, the cheese, and the sausage. I could taste it, without even putting it my mouth. Still I managed to hang tough and stick with the fish. Someday I will be normal, I told myself, and I will be eating that pizza just like all of the other people. I just had to hang on. Sure.

When I got home after the party, it turned out that the story was only half finished. As I lay in bed, thinking about my "success", I found myself losing control. I couldn't get food off my mind. I still wanted that damn pizza.

As if in a trance, I got back up out of bed and went down to the kitchen. I had probably the worst binge of my life. I ate everything I could find. I consumed everything in the refrigerator—inhaled it—might be a better description. I think I even ripped a few cupboard doors off their hinges. I was consumed with a barrage of emotions:

Self-hate: why couldn't I just be normal like everybody else?

Regret: I still wanted that pizza.

Shame: I didn't really belong at that party with my friends, at least not until I was normal.

Embarrassment: I must have looked pretty foolish eating fish in a pizza restaurant.

Sadness: I didn't want to be so fat and ugly. Life was passing me by.

Then, as I devoured food from the refrigerator, I began to feel guilt about my current behavior. Now I'd done it. I'd wrecked everything. I'd probably already gained back the 20 pounds I'd worked so hard to lose. I really was worthless. Instead of going to Weight Watchers next Monday with a great success story, I was probably going to be too ashamed to show up at all. I would have to climb on that scale and see how badly things had gone, and try for forgiveness and understanding from the instructor. Well, probably not. More than likely, I would just skip the whole thing. For now, I might as well enjoy my binge with all of that hell waiting for me.

I eventually was so stuffed that I couldn't eat any more. Did I get back on the diet the next day? Of course not. What was the point? I'd already blown it. And, as you might expect, I didn't go back to Weight Watchers, at least not right away. I'd have to wait until I lost the weight that I'd gained, so I could put things right again.

As usual, I waited to "re-join" Weight Watchers the next time it made sense. After the holidays, I think. To this day, I wonder what would have happened if I'd just eaten the pizza.

The Thin Person Paradigm

I've included the pizza story to demonstrate the fat paradigm and I hope that you will have recognized at least some of the distorted thinking present. I thought of myself as different from the others at the party. They were thin—I was fat. Therefore, we should behave differently. I wanted to be on "their side of the table", but I didn't feel that I was. It was necessary for me to fake it in some manner just to be there at all.

Nobody else at the party was fat, at least not like I was. Everybody ate from the same pizza. Nobody got fat from eating the pizza. Why couldn't I eat the same pizza? What was the difference?

Now, you might argue that I was dieting and that eating the pizza would destroy the magic of the diet. However, if I were to behave the same as a thin person, wouldn't I look just like a thin person? Wasn't that what I was truly after anyway? I just wanted to be normal and live like everybody else. I didn't realize that I already was.

The reason that I was fat wasn't that I ate pizza and that it affected me differently, the reason that I was fat was that I ate *more* than the thin people did. If I was brutally honest with myself, I knew that to be true. Even though I spent a lot of energy trying to convince myself that I was somehow afflicted with a different metabolism, I knew deep down inside that I ate a ton of food. I didn't do it in public and I denied it to myself, but I ate all the time. I ate for any reason I could find.

I pretended very hard that I didn't. I would go to McDonald's at lunch, order a large (but not too large) amount of food so that I wouldn't embarrass myself in front of the kid taking my order. Then I'd eat it, drive next door to Burger King, and order more. All this so that nobody could see me overeating. I could honestly claim to be eating just like everybody else; the difference was that I was just doing it all the time.

I had a binge anytime I tried to restrict my eating. I don't know if I was rebelling or simply proving to myself that I was worthless and couldn't do it. I do know that it seemed to make me feel better. It eventually washed away any emotions that I was feeling, except for the lingering guilt and self-disgust, and

I could quickly get rid of those feelings by planning my next diet. I was sure things would be better soon.

It never dawned on me that I really was just like everybody else. Instead of behaving like a fat person trying to be thin, I should think like a thin person and not worry about it.

What in the world is wrong with going to a pizza party and eating pizza with friends? What would be different if I got thin first and then went to the party? Would that pizza have affected me any differently? Would I still have chosen the broiled fish, or would my metabolism now be different and pizza would be okay, just as it was for the thin people? I don't think so. Nothing would be different. And that is the point: Nothing *is* different.

I didn't need permission from Weight Watchers to eat pizza. I didn't need permission from anybody. It was my life and I needed to live it like I chose. I sure didn't need anybody to tell me what to eat. I already knew all there was to know about that.

In reality, there is no food that will make you fat!

Even if I ate a lot of pizza, simply listening to my body telling me when it was hungry again would have taken care of it. Rather than listening to my emotions demanding to be suppressed, I probably would have eaten less food for a while without even thinking about it. There would be no harm in having eaten the pizza, even if I overdid it a little.

Nutrition in a Nutshell: Write It Down

As easy and straightforward as that all sounds, there are still problems to be dealt with. Most fat people don't have a clue when they're hungry and when they're not. Their behavior is such that it is unrealistic to expect that they will simply begin to behave in a "normal" fashion after years of self-abuse and self-punishment. Something needs to change, but it isn't diet; it's behavior.

The Nutrition Cornerstone is really the easiest of the four, or at least it may seem that way at first. It is more about unlearning than learning. The idea is to eat what you want when you want, but no matter what you eat, you must write it in the nutrition section of your journal. Sound simple? Just wait. I'll bet you will have no trouble writing down the things that you feel are "acceptable" foods, but will have a terrible time writing down anything that is "bad". The pen won't move across the page or you will "forget" that you ate something. Denial is not so easy to push aside.

As we learned in the journaling section, there is tremendous power in writing. The ability to write is one of the most recently developed in the human skill set, and we apparently make use of parts of the brain that cause us to process information differently than simply thinking about something, or even talking about it. As you write what you've eaten each day, things begin to happen to your behavior. Patterns become apparent and subtle changes start to occur.

One of my old habits was to sneak off to a secluded vending machine at work every day at about 3:00 and eat three or four candy bars. I made sure that nobody saw me and of course told no one about my indulgence. However, once I began writing that down every day, things started to change. At first, I couldn't remember exactly how many candy bars I had eaten, so I'd have to guess. But that made me want to write the exact amount down, so the next day I'd consciously count them as I ate them, so that I could be more honest in the journal. Something about seeing my behavior spelled out in writing, by my own hand, caused me to think further about what I was doing.

After a few days of writing down all of the food that I was eating, I would notice changes in what I craved. Even though I was well aware of the candy bars, at some level I was still in denial. Writing it down began to flush that behavior more out into the open. I started to wish that I wasn't doing that every day. I began to realize that this was something that tended to happen about 3:00 and I would get curious about that. Could it wait until 4:00? Could I have two candy bars instead of three? Could I make myself eat five bars even if I wanted less?

I would experiment and somehow my mind and my intentions started to get a handle on my behavior. Usually around 3:00, for reasons that I never became clear about, I realized that I would feel angry. I don't know if it was work related, or if it was something that went back to my childhood. I just felt frustration about that time every day and I didn't like it. Eating made it go away, at least for a while.

After a few weeks of this, *something* made me want to stop. I didn't know everything wrong about the way I ate, but certainly I knew that raiding the vending machine daily wasn't what I needed to be doing.

One day, I just didn't do it. I anticipated the candy bar cravings and they came, but I didn't follow my impulse to binge. As I resisted, I immediately felt a feeling of anger inside me, although I didn't know about what.

The anger grew and I felt frantic. What was this feeling I was having? How bad was it going to get? Could I really resist my chocolate ritual? I remember that I felt so angry that I decided to leave work early. By the time I got home, I was feeling tremendous anger, but I still didn't know why. I wanted to eat to stop the anger. There was a pile of wood sitting in the garage. I knew that I had to let the feeling out, or I would go into the kitchen and binge. I picked up a hammer (I know this sounds bizarre) and began to whack on some wood. I let whatever I was feeling come out by smashing that poor log to pieces. I thought I was loosing my mind, but it stopped after a couple of minutes and I began to feel somewhat relieved. I didn't know what I was mad about and I didn't know why, but it really didn't matter. The feelings had to go some-where and I was tired of having them go into my mouth in the form of food and then to be carried around in the form of fat.

It was not that things instantly got better after that, but I do feel it was a clear turning point for me. I would still occasionally want to visit the vending machine, but never with the intensity that I had felt before. I knew that there was something else going on besides hunger and, more importantly, that it was getting in the way of my intentions. Just acknowledging that I was trying to "eat away" an emotion, made me more eager to express that feeling rather than avoid it.

By writing everything down that I ate, my journal let me look at life differ-ently. What was I feeling when I ate? What had happened that made feel that way? Was I punishing myself for something? Was I celebrating something? Was I hurt or offended? Or ignored? What was I really feeling that I wanted to hide in a food binge?

Don't Dwell On the "Why"

The "why" of our behavior can be quite fascinating and many things will be revealed to you if you let them, but that really isn't the point. I have met many people who already seem quite in touch with the "why" of their self-abusive behavior, but still are unable to get a handle on "what" they are doing.

The power of writing down everything that you eat is that it gives you a handle on the "what", not so much on the "why". Even if you understand the roots of your actions, you still must change them if you genuinely want to change your life.

If you begin to see the specifics of what you are doing, you can lay out a plan to change it. You can see how it conflicts with your overall goal, and if you are truly clear on that larger goal, you can begin to change what you do to begin to reach it.

When you seem stuck and you are unable to do what it is that you feel is appropriate, that is the time to examine the "why". Take a look at just what you are feeling when you "blow it". What is going on inside you? Look over the list of feelings at the back of this book and see if any of them ring a bell when you feel yourself slipping. Is it sadness, or anger? Are you scared or happy?

The journal will begin to give you a new perspective on yourself. It will make you feel a sense of awareness and therefore a sense of control over your actions.

Food Agreements

As you master the power of the agreement, you probably will want to use it to reshape your eating habits. Most people that I have met using the Cornerstone approach immediately attack their eating habits with agreements about what they "won't" eat, and then fail.

It is tempting to try to solve your eating compulsions with an attack of agreements. On occasion, this may be appropriate, but be very careful. For fat people, eating is by far the most delicate behavior in their lives and the least straightforward.

Agreeing to eat less is like agreeing to breathe less. Our desire to eat is a biological need, just like breathing, and we are just about as likely to succeed in consuming less food as we would be in consuming less air. Our bodies will tell us what to eat just like they tell us how hard to breathe. It is a function of our activities, not something that can be decided in advance.

The other Cornerstones will cause changes in your need for food. As you reduce stress, become more physically fit, and get a better handle on your feelings through the other three Cornerstones, your dysfunctional need to overeat should diminish. Follow your needs and don't worry so much about what you are eating, as long as you are honestly able to write everything that you eat in your journal.

Remember that it is better to agree to "do" something, than to "not do" something. Even as I found my desire to binge eat decreasing, I still had many bad habits left that needed to be addressed. It was in dealing with these bad habits that I made most of my food agreements.

As I've mentioned before, one of my ongoing problems was that when I came home in the evenings, I would immediately head toward the refrigerator and begin eating. I wouldn't change clothes, I wouldn't take my tie off, and I would barely set my briefcase down before I started grabbing food. Before I knew it, I would have consumed much more than I really needed and I hadn't even thought about dinner.

My first thought was to make an agreement not to raid the refrigerator when I walked in the door, but that left me feeling empty and it was a difficult agreement to keep in that it was an agreement "not" to do something. I revised the agreement to agree that I would change clothes before I began eating. I was free to raid the refrigerator, but I at least needed to put on more comfortable clothes before doing it.

This approach worked much better. I wasn't restricting or eliminating anything, I was simply adding my own controls around the situation. I could eat like crazy if I wanted to; I just had to have a handle on myself before I started.

The effect was amazing. The simple 10-minute delay in the daily binge was a manageable goal. I wasn't fighting with myself about whether I should or shouldn't eat; I was just agreeing to alter the circumstances slightly. By the time I'd changed clothes, the desire to overeat was much more in control. I would still eat a snack, but it wasn't loaded with the guilt that drove me to eat even more than I wanted. I was hungry when I got home and I satisfied the hunger. Adding a measure of personal control to the situation carried forward and I would usually be able to stop before I'd eaten a tremendous amount of food and spoiled the evening.

Delay Tactics, Turning Into the Skid, and the Binge

Most people that I have met in the Cornerstone classes have trouble with binge eating. In my experience, it is the most difficult area for the fat person to get a handle on. It is as if a trance like state consumes us, and by the time we recover from this pleasant but damaging behavior, we are stuffed to the bursting point and loaded with guilt, shame, and all sorts of self-hate.

The binge can be quite dangerous in some situations. I remember meeting a man several years ago at an Overeaters Anonymous meeting who had actually once eaten so much during a binge that his stomach had burst. Think about that. Could it possibly have been hunger driving him to eat that much?

Hardly. When the binge starts, the demons are back in control trying desperately to ruin our best intentions.

When I feel myself losing control, I have a standing agreement that I will first grab my journal and try my best to write down my feelings. As I've gotten better about tapping into what I'm feeling and letting it flow out of my pen, rather than into my mouth, the craving is greatly diminished, if not altogether eliminated.

I don't try to slam on the brakes and eliminate the binge. That tends to cause an even more severe binge. The analogy I like to use is to think about what we learned back in high school driver's education class: When the car begins to skid out of control, turn into the skid, not away from it. Never slam on the brakes, because it will cause a further loss of control. The idea is to move with the skid, not away from it, until the wheels of the car are aligned with the direction of the car, and then to gently guide the car back to were we want it to go.

This is the way to handle a binge. When we feel the skid starting, rather than fight it, roll with it. Don't start arguing with yourself about it; have a plan of attack ready to get a handle on the situation and bring yourself back under control.

For example, agree to a 10-minute journal session before eating and then eat what you want. Those 10 minutes of writing might give you some real clues as to what is causing the binge in the first place. There is a good chance that your unconscious mind will allow you this 10-minute interlude if it knows that it is only a temporary delay, not a cancellation of the binge. By taking that 10-minute journal delay, you are inserting a piece of yourself into the "skid" and giving yourself a little bit of an "out" by retaining just a hint of control of the situation.

Even if the binge is as severe as it would have been without the 10-minute journal session, like a scientist gathering data, you will have collected at least a clue as to what is sending you out of control so that you can recover more quickly and possibly lay out a plan to avoid the situation in the future.

Use your journal to work backwards through the day's events to see if you can find a trigger. Was it work related, spouse related, children related? Did you fail at something? Were you disappointed in yourself in some way? Angry? Sad? It is particularly useful to scan the feelings list at the back of this book before the binge, to see if you can correctly identify what it is you are feeling besides hunger as you start the binge. Then after the binge, see if you can find the roots of that feeling in some event during the day. It may have happened hours ago, or it may have just occurred.

As the pieces of the puzzle come together, the mystery may begin to reveal itself to you. It may take many binges before you start to understand. Don't expect miracles. Just continue to "turn into the skid" whenever you get in trouble, get a handle on yourself as quickly as you can and get your car back on the road. No matter how much you eat during a binge, it can't possibly be enough to undo the progress you've made overall in establishing a new paradigm.

The Reset Button

Create an image of a big red button labeled "reset" somewhere inside your head. Burn this image into your mind! Whenever you have started down the path of eating something that you would rather not be eating, remember this picture. There is a reset button inside your mind. All you have to do is push it and you will stop, right then. Just because you've started eating something, doesn't mean that you have to finish it. You can quickly disable the behavior just by pressing the reset button. It will "re-boot" your mental computer and give you a fresh start.

The simple concept of the reset button made all of the difference for me. I used to think in terms of weeks when I thought about overeating. If I'd "blown it", I would feel that I must wait until next Monday to get going start over, or at least wait until tomorrow. This day was lost, so I might as well enjoy it and start again on a better day. In the mean time, I should eat like crazy, because soon I wouldn't be able to. Once I got back on the wagon, I'm wasn't going to be able to eat like this, so once again it was time to indulge in yet another *Last Supper!* After that, I could think about getting control of my life.

The reality is there is no beginning and no end. If you want a better life, it has already started. There is no tomorrow. Any improvement in your lifestyle must include behaviors to handle the rough spots, because there will always be rough spots. The healthier you get, the more confusing the rough spots will become, so get used to it.

There is no magic starting line that you must wait to cross; you've already crossed it when you started reading this book. In reality, you crossed it the day you were born. It is all part of life and there is only one way out, which I doubt that you are eager to experience; at least I hope not!

So, as you start into something that you know you would rather not, stop. Reset. Right then. Don't worry about what you've done; worry about what you are doing. The sooner the better. You're not on a diet; eating that candy bar (or whatever) isn't ruining anything. But if it represents something that you don't want to do, then stop.

That candy bar isn't going to make you fat. Your overall lifestyle will determine your size and wellness. The big picture is what matters.

With a little practice, I was able to visualize that reset button in the middle of a binge. It became an icon of self-control. I could push it and the binge would stop. It was that simple. I came to know that I was in control. I knew what I wanted out of life and I knew that this binge wasn't a part of it. It really is quite simple when you look at it through a different paradigm.

Ironically, the greatest strides come when we slip and then gain control of a disastrous situation. Much more progress comes from learning how to recover from a disaster than from managing to avoid it. There is simply no way we can structure our lives not to have problems; it can't be done. It makes much more sense to develop tools to deal with problems than to waste so much time trying to avoid them. We need the confidence that comes from the knowledge that we will be able to deal with unforeseen problems.

You are going to overeat. You are going to lose control. Plan for it, deal with it, and then get on with it. The reset button is your spare tire. It won't be used in pleasant situations, but sooner or later, you will need it. And if it doesn't work, that is okay too. You're still on your journey whether you like it or not. You'll find a solution if you keep looking.

If you adopt that slightly different outlook on things, tremendous changes can happen. The Nutrition Cornerstone is more about unlearning than learning. We have filled our minds with distorted concepts that keep getting us in trouble. We must look at life through a new paradigm. We have become people that are living the life that we want and are no longer slaves to the ideas of others about food.

Forget the Scale

As you throw out your concept of **THE DIET,** you might want to throw out your scale as well. Nothing adds to the confusion of getting healthier more than climbing on top of a scale and letting it tell us whether or not we are succeeding. Just as we know what to eat and when, we also know if we are doing it and we don't need some external device to tell us.

The scale frequently gives wrong signals. It can be discouraging when it should be encouraging. Not many things are as maddening as feeling good about how well we've been eating, but not getting immediate results on the scale.

More importantly, I would hope by now that you are beginning to realize that it isn't weight loss that you seek, but a completely new and rewarding life, a life that you've chosen for yourself. That new life will produce results long before any scale can.

You won't need anybody or anything to tell you when you are making progress, you will already know.

Using a scale to monitor progress smacks of having a goal weight—a future point in time where you will be "fixed". That never happens. There is no starting line further down the road that you will cross and life will begin; you've already crossed it. So forget about how much you weigh. Work on improving how you live.

People always ask me how long it took to lose my fat and I really don't know. One of my first agreements was only to weigh myself once a month. And then, I pretty much stopped that altogether. I knew that I was doing what I wanted to do, and it didn't really matter how quickly I was losing weight. Losing weight was only a by-product of what it was that I really wanted in life. There was no need to track it.

It can be surprisingly difficult to stop weighing yourself, to give up looking to an external source for acknowledgment of your success. It is too much a part of our culture to discard, but the scale can be a good source of agreement making by delaying climbing onto it for a day, or a week, or a month—whatever you can handle. Think like the naturally thin person that you are. There is no need to fret about small "ups and downs" on the scale; everything will be fine in the end.

If you truly want a measure of your progress, have the doctor or a health club calculate the percentage of body fat that you have. It is an interesting process. As I got more into long distance running, I increased the amount of muscle that I had and so did my weight. I would have been most discouraged if I'd seen my weight climbing with all the exercise I was now doing.

However, nothing that elaborate is really necessary. You will know when you are leading the life you want. You don't need body fat calculations or even a tape measure to tell you about it. You'll know. The real trick is to look into yourself to determine how you are doing, to look past all of the denial, and perform your own reality check.

The "1 to 10" Scale of Hunger

A great device to help tune into your true level of hunger is the "1 to 10" scale. Imagine a gauge inside you that rates your current level of "fullness", similar to the fuel gauge on your car. A reading of 1 indicates such incredibly intense hunger that you would eat almost anything to make the pain go away—say you'd be willing to scoop up a handful of dirt if nothing else were available. A reading of 10 is that post-Thanksgiving bloat feeling where you have to have someone help you onto the couch and unbutton your clothes before they rip open. A reading of 5 is exactly in the middle, no sense of hunger, and no sense of fullness. A level 5 would feel like you had no stomach at all. Ideally, you would be at a 5 at all times, but of course, this is impossible. As you expend energy, you will always need new fuel to keep going.

It is usually impossible to just fill back up exactly to a level 5 without occasionally going over to a 6 or 7, but to go beyond that requires some sort of abusive eating or conscious choice.

The point of balance is the level 5. A level 5 reading will tune your system to your current set point, and you will find yourself eating just enough to stay right there. As your level of stress drops, your emotional balance stabilizes, and your level of fitness increases, your set point will lower and you will actually be tuning into a new setting without realizing it. So, a level 5 reading on your hunger scale will actually cause you to lose fat until you've reached your new set point.

When I was losing fat, I tried to keep my level at about a 4. It wasn't really necessary, but that faint feeling of hunger was a constant reminder that I was right on track and in tune with my goals in life and I truly welcomed it. I liked to keep just a slight, distant feeling of hunger, but nothing that would send me over the edge. I actually grew to enjoy that feeling. It felt light and energizing in contrast to the stuffed feeling I was used to. But a level 5 is all you need to get your body in tune with itself.

You should continually assess your hunger level. What is it right now? Whenever it is anything below level 4, eat something soon. If you drop down to levels below that, you are asking for trouble. Very quickly, you will find yourself losing control and very possibly starting a binge. When you get much above a level 6, you are heading into guilt territory and that could trigger a binge as well. Your goal is to keep the reading right between 4 and 6 and to do whatever is necessary to keep it there. This is the range of sanity and you will be much more likely to keep agreements and feel good about yourself if you stay in the 4 to 6 range.

When you do eat more than is necessary and go up to maybe a 7 or 8 during a special occasion, don't worry about it. As long as you keep tuning into the level reading to determine when and how much should eat next, you'll be fine. If you have an unusually large lunch, for example, you won't be as hungry when dinner comes. It may be 10 o'clock at night before your level gets back down to a 4 or 5, and that will be the proper time to eat. Your body is quite capable of telling you what it needs and when. If you are like most fat people, you've just long ago stopped listening to it, but it will be happy to tell you all that you need to know. No diets, scales, or doses of guilt are necessary.

This is the secret of thin people—they eat when they are hungry, and they eat what they are hungry for. What a novel concept! And now for the best news of all: you are just like they are. Forget about metabolism and age and bone structure and whatever else you've been telling yourself is the reason that you are different from thin people. You already are a thin person.

Vitamins

I have to admit I've bought into the idea of vitamin supplements. There is no reason that I know of that we shouldn't take advantage of the technology available to us in the form of vitamins. The only harm that I can possibly think of is some of the ridiculous claims made by vitamin manufacturers about promoting weight loss through a supplement. That isn't going to happen, but I have come to believe that it is worthwhile to ensure that I'm getting a good dose of vitamins at all times. It is quite possible that some food cravings come from vitamin deficiency as our bodies try desperately to find a source of the needed nutrient. What can the harm be in making sure we get a good balance?

As I became healthier, I found myself feeling better about going to health food stores and listening to the various claims about exotic vitamins and foods. I never completely believed what I heard, but it seemed to add to the adventure of food and served to keep my mind open to new ideas. Just striving for a healthier lifestyle and creating a new level of awareness seemed valuable.

Nutrition and a Sense of Adventure

I've reached a point where I constantly seek out new foods that I've never tried before—the more exotic, the better. This is yet another area where acquiring a taste for adventure is a key element. Sometimes, new things turn out to be awful, but so what?

I've gotten in the habit of trying to find new restaurants that serve a cuisine that I've never tried before. Vegetarian, Indian, Oriental, whatever, it doesn't matter. The adventure is the key to continually expanding my food consciousness. Fat people tend to have terribly limited food repertoires, even though they claim to love food. They eat the same things over and over, as if in a trance. Trying new things is way of breaking out of that mold. What difference does it make if something turns out to be terrible? Throw it out and try something else.

Whenever I've traveled to a foreign country, I've tried to find things that I've never eaten before. I didn't worry about how nutritious they were; I just wanted to make sure that I experienced something that I wouldn't have had the opportunity to sample otherwise.

Think of your most favorite food. Now, realize that you wouldn't know that it *was* your favorite if you'd never tried it. Moreover, if you expand on that concept, how do you know that there isn't something even better lurking in some exotic restaurant if you don't take a chance?

Pay attention to which foods are the most satisfying and how long the feeling of satisfaction lasts. I realized, for example, that high fiber foods really worked best for me. They were the most filling and the feeling lasted the longest. High fiber kept things "moving" through me, adding to that overall feeling of cleansing that I feel when I perspire heavily during a workout. If I ate a lot of meat, on the other hand, the reverse happened. I began to feel bloated. I found myself naturally gravitating towards higher fiber foods by choice rather than by forcing myself to change my eating habits. But that is just me and you probably will be different!

I began getting curious about healthier foods naturally, but really only after most of my fat was gone. It came more from a sense of adventure than anything else. I started wondering what could be done with tofu, or what was behind the thinking of vegetarians. One of my favorite restaurants is a vegetarian restaurant and I get a real thrill out of going there to see what they've managed to do without meat, but I've never really attempted to get into vegetarianism. It is just a curiosity to me, like any other type of food.

Use Your Journal to Identify Patterns

After enough tracking of what you eat, you'll probably begin to notice that certain foods appeal to you under certain circumstances and can be a leading indicator of troubles down the road.

I've noticed, for example, that when I crave sweets, I'm angry with myself, for one reason or another. I've been disappointed by something and somehow sweet candy elevates my mood, but only temporarily. It is usually a sign that I need to get working in my journal and sort out the real issue.

When I'm stressed out, fatty foods seem to appeal more. It is almost as if they are calming in some way. That is a sign that a little more work in the Stress Reduction Cornerstone is needed.

I also make a very rough guess at the number of calories for each food item I've eaten. I round off to the nearest 100 calories and write that in my journal next to each item of food that I've eaten. At the end of the day, I total the calories just to see where I was for the day.

I don't try to restrict the number of calories that I eat. I just eat when I'm hungry, but I do take note of when the total appears to be climbing as another leading indicator that things might be starting to come apart in my life. The solution always lies in the other three Cornerstones.

It is worthwhile to be aware of the rough number of calories in a given food item, but only a rough count. For example, I count any apple as 100 calories and any candy bar as 300, and that is good enough. I don't weigh or measure, I just take an educated guess and go with that. Most fat people are walking calorie dictionaries and can recite the exact number of calories in just about any food. That is unnecessary. Most of us eat pretty much the same things over and over each week, and learning the caloric count of those base foods will be more than enough information for our purposes.

Lately, counting fat or carbohydrate grams has become fashionable, but I don't pay much attention to that. Experiment with it if it appeals to you, but don't do it in an effort to restrict your fat intake. Just see it leads you and make adjustments as needed. I prefer calories simply because it gives a better overall sense of quantity of food, not just a measure of a specific component like fat or protein.

I want to stress that the point of estimating calories is only to give a rough indicator of where you are going with your food intake on a given day, not to restrict it in any way. Some days you will need more and other days you will need less. You are only looking for warning signs and leading indicators. You are not dieting. Your only guide to how much you eat should be the "1 to 10" scale of hunger, not trying to keep your calorie count below a certain point. If you are craving more food, figure out why but don't fight the urge, it is quite natural.

Remember that you are a thin person and you can eat what you want when you want. You are only trying to become *aware* of what you eat.

Support from the Other Cornerstones

I suspect that to the long-time dieter, all of this "eat what you want" stuff sounds like nonsense. The idea that we should naturally follow our eating instincts is probably quite frightening if nothing else, like walking a tightrope without a net. It will take some unlearning.

However, don't forget that you won't be doing this in a vacuum! You are doing activities from the other three Cornerstones that are going to have subtle but definite effects on your level of hunger and improve your outlook on life in general.

The difference between the Cornerstones and a traditional diet is that the Cornerstones cause changes from the inside, not the outside. Their purpose is not to restrict your behavior to match somebody else's idea of how you should be living your life.

Always Forgive Yourself

A final word about guilt and shame is probably in order. When you find yourself experiencing either of those two feelings, particularly with respect to what you've eaten, get the journal out and sort it out.

The most important habit you can develop is to be able to forgive yourself, no matter what. Guilt and shame are simply ways of punishing ourselves so that we can clear the slate and then do whatever we did all over again.

Guilt and shame are not simple emotions. Nobody was born being able to feel either guilt or shame. Someone had to teach us how to feel them. If we had to learn them, we can unlearn them, which will go a long way towards correcting our behavior.

Instead of feeling guilty about something that you've eaten or done, why not figure out some way so that you won't repeat the crime, rather than beating yourself up in some form of punishment? The deed is done; get on with it!

And, since you won't be making rules about what you eat, you won't be setting up rules to be broken and feel badly about, right? If you handle the Nutrition Cornerstone correctly, there will be no opportunity to feel guilty or shameful. You are in tune with your needs. Case closed.

Suggestions

- Throw away your scale. Use your resting pulse or body fat measurement as your gauge of success.

- Write everything you eat (good or bad) in your journal.

- When you are deciding if you are able to eat something, ask yourself if you've ever seen a thin person eating it. If so, it's okay to eat.

- Before eating, decide how hungry you are on the "1 to 10" scale. While you are eating, try to decide how the hunger rating is changing.

- Use your journal to associate your emotions with the times you feel hungry.

- When you feel the need to binge, try waiting a few minutes first to see what emotions emerge.

- Don't fight binges, try to "turn into the skid", rather than slamming on the brakes. No matter how crazy you feel, you are still in control.

- If you start a binge, remember that it's okay to stop. You haven't ruined anything.

- Use the "Reset Button" to visualize getting back on track.

- After you've had a binge, get in the habit of forgiving yourself immediately and then moving on.

- Remember that you don't have to wait until the beginning of a week, a day, or even an hour to get back on track.

- Try being hungry for a little while and see if the world ends.

- Acquire a taste for adventure!

Favorite Excuses

- I don't have the time to eat healthy meals. Besides, they keep changing the rules about what healthy food is.

- I always forget what I've eaten and therefore can't write it down.

- I never forget what I've eaten and therefore don't need to write it down.

- I don't know what to eat.

- My metabolism won't let me lose weight anyway. I don't eat anymore than anyone else; I'm just meant to be fat.

- I can't stop binge eating.

- I'm going to start on Monday.

- I get headaches (or faint) when I'm hungry.

- I'm addicted to chocolate (or whatever else).

- I'm exercising enough so that I can eat whatever I want.

- Certain foods make me fat.

- I only write down the good things I'm eating.

- I can't socialize or go to restaurants until I'm thin.

- So-and-so can have whatever they want and I can't.

- I think the world should accept me as I am.

- My family won't eat the foods that I need to eat.

- I heard about a new diet that is *really* supposed to work.

- I only have time for fast food.

- The cafeteria only serves fattening food.

Add your favorite excuses here!

- _____
- _____
- _____
- _____
- _____
- _____
- _____
- _____
- _____
- _____
- _____
- _____

8

Putting It All Together

It is so important that you realize that each of the Cornerstones is equally important and will build support for the others. It doesn't work to pick only the ones that are easy and ignore the rest.

Different people find that different Cornerstones are more difficult. That is how it should be because we are all at different places in our lives and have gotten there following different paths. The Cornerstone that gives you the most frustration will inevitably be the most valuable.

Much more is learned from our mistakes than from our successes. The things that we already know how to do will only produce the results that we already have. If we want more, we must do something differently or do something new. Rarely will we get it right the first time, or probably even the second. Mistakes should be welcomed, not feared.

Is it realistic to expect our lives to change if we aren't willing to change ourselves? There is a big difference between changing our lives and wanting our lives to change.

The Fitness Cornerstone will improve our physical selves. It will shatter the notion that we are somehow physically less capable or different from the rest of the world. Of course, we are all different and all have different levels of abilities, but there is no one who can't move further along the path of physical. This is as true for the Olympic Athlete as it is for the Couch Potato. The only real measure of our own performance is our previous performance. It is not valid to compare ourselves with others.

The Stress Reduction Cornerstone will allow us to feel more in control of ourselves and will help eliminate the stress created by making changes in our lives. Anything new generates stress, good or bad. Most of us are stressed out already and adding the Cornerstone infrastructure is going to add even more stress. The Stress Reduction Cornerstone provides an outlet for that stress, in a natural and productive way. No more need to kick the dog (or other loved ones); we have a new tool in our tool kit.

The Nutrition Cornerstone mainly serves to create a heightened level of food consciousness, nothing more. It is not about dieting or restricting ourselves in any way. It is about reconnecting with our natural needs for nutrition and learning what that means in our day-to-day life.

The Journal Keeping Cornerstone ties it all together. It gives a daily record of all of our Cornerstone activities. It provides a place to connect with our feelings in a positive and useful way, rather than eating them in the form of a binge. It is a place to plan and provides a tool to break through whatever denial we may have that is keeping us stuck in the past.

But don't forget the paradigm shift! I have seen people do a nice job with all Four Cornerstones but make little progress in general. If you aren't clear about where you are going, if you are denying what it is that you really want out of life, don't expect any real changes to occur. You certainly will feel better if you adopt the Four Cornerstones as part of your lifestyle. If you haven't gotten clear on where it is that you want to be in life, you will probably only experience a moderate improvement.

Paradigm shifts are an ongoing part of living. Sometimes we call them mid-life crises, or sometimes they come in the form of a personal revelation or an epiphany, but everybody has them and they can be quite disturbing. Whatever goals you may have identified for yourself now might turn out to be completely wrong later on. That is as it should be. It is unlikely that you will get it right the first time. The only point is that you must want something different, or you wouldn't be reading this book.

Make sure that you use the Cornerstones to look past the issue of fat. *Fat is nothing but a symptom of a paradigm that is misaligned with personal goals.* You must seek out what it is that you really want and then develop a new way of thinking about yourself to obtain that goal.

Once you have experienced one paradigm shift, the subsequent ones become much easier. Once you know that you can change the way you look at things, you will become much more open to new possibilities down the road. You will begin to understand the relativity of belief systems.

People who attempt to get through life without ever changing their way of thinking about things seem to wind up old and grouchy. Their way of dealing with life has stopped working, but they refuse to accept that and instead demand that the rest of the world adapt to them. On the other hand, people who have learned to adapt and adjust tend to be much happier and enjoy new adventures throughout their entire lives and have a much more pleasant outlook in general. Which would you prefer?

The Cornerstones are very much a personal journey. What works for one person might fail for another. You must be the judge and jury of what it right for you. Only you know what you are seeking and only you can make it happen. But, whatever you do, remember to enjoy the adventure. Bon voyage!

Appendix A

Feeling Identification Prompt List

The following is a list of feelings to use to in assessing your current state of mind. Scan through the list and see what best represents what you are feeling at this moment. Use it as a beginning to make an entry in your journal—if only to write that particular feeling down—and see what comes next. The feelings are grouped very roughly by category. This is only a small subset of all of things that you might be feeling at any given moment. It is meant only to prompt you into looking further into your feelings. Try to find the exact "shade" of the emotion you are experiencing. Categorizing feelings can be extremely useful in the journal process. You may not be able to figure out why you are feeling the way you are, but knowing exactly what you are feeling is the more important issue.

Space is provided at the end of the list to add any additional feelings you might identify that might be useful in the future for subsequent journaling.

Sad

- Lonely
- Depressed
- Ashamed
- Bored
- Guilty

- Miserable
- Inadequate
- Inferior
- Stupid
- Sleepy
- Apathetic
- Listless
- Bashful

Mad

- Angry
- Rage
- Hostile
- Frustrated
- Furious
- Hateful
- Critical
- Skeptical
- Irritated
- Hurt
- Jealous
- Selfish

Scared

- Insecure
- Anxious
- Nervous

- Apprehensive
- Embarrassed
- Humiliated
- Rejected
- Helpless
- Confused
- Discouraged
- Bewildered
- Insignificant
- Submissive
- Weak
- Foolish

Powerful

- Confident
- Important
- Proud
- Appreciated
- Respected
- Worthwhile
- Valuable
- Intelligent
- Satisfied
- Hopeful
- Faithful

Happy

- Ecstatic
- Exhilarated
- Blissful
- Cheerful
- Amused
- Energetic
- Delighted
- Extravagant
- Stimulated
- Sexy
- Excited
- Fascinated
- Playful
- Creative
- Aware
- Daring

Calm

- Peaceful
- Relaxed
- Serene
- Thoughtful
- Intimate
- Content
- Loving

- Trusting
- Responsive
- Nurturing
- Thankful
- Pensive

Hungry?

Add additional feelings here!

- _____
- _____
- _____
- _____
- _____
- _____
- _____
- _____
- _____
- _____
- _____
- _____

APPENDIX B

Sample Journal

This section contains sample journal layouts for a month of journaling to get you started, but don't stop at the end of a month. *Start today, even if it isn't Monday!* You can use these pages for your initial journal, or may want to keep your journal in a separate book. Some people use a computer software program to allow them to password protect their writing and to make it more searchable. You will probably need to adjust your journaling strategy as time goes by, but whatever you do, make the journal be your basis for all of your Cornerstone efforts. The information and support it will provide is endless and it is fundamental to the Cornerstone methodology.

Date:	
Fitness:	**Stress Reduction:**
Resting Pulse Rate:	
Nutrition:	

Journal:

Date:	
Fitness:	**Stress Reduction:**
Resting Pulse Rate:	
Nutrition:	
Journal:	

Date:	
Fitness:	**Stress Reduction:**
Resting Pulse Rate:	
Nutrition:	
Journal:	

Date:	
Fitness:	Stress Reduction:
Resting Pulse Rate:	
Nutrition:	
Journal:	

Date:	
Fitness:	**Stress Reduction:**
Resting Pulse Rate:	
Nutrition:	
Journal:	

Date:	
Fitness:	**Stress Reduction:**
Resting Pulse Rate:	
Nutrition:	

Journal:

Date:	
Fitness:	**Stress Reduction:**
Resting Pulse Rate:	
Nutrition:	
Journal:	

Date:	
Fitness:	**Stress Reduction:**
Resting Pulse Rate:	
Nutrition:	
Journal:	

Date:	
Fitness:	**Stress Reduction:**
Resting Pulse Rate:	
Nutrition:	
Journal:	

Date:	
Fitness:	**Stress Reduction:**
Resting Pulse Rate:	
Nutrition:	

Journal:

Date:	
Fitness:	**Stress Reduction:**
Resting Pulse Rate:	
Nutrition:	
Journal:	

Date:	
Fitness:	**Stress Reduction:**
Resting Pulse Rate:	
Nutrition:	

Journal:

Date:	
Fitness:	**Stress Reduction:**
Resting Pulse Rate:	
Nutrition:	
Journal:	

Date:	
Fitness:	**Stress Reduction:**
Resting Pulse Rate:	
Nutrition:	
Journal:	

Date:	
Fitness:	**Stress Reduction:**
Resting Pulse Rate:	
Nutrition:	
Journal:	

Date:	
Fitness:	**Stress Reduction:**
Resting Pulse Rate:	
Nutrition:	
Journal:	

Date:	
Fitness:	**Stress Reduction:**
Resting Pulse Rate:	
Nutrition:	
Journal:	

Date:	
Fitness:	**Stress Reduction:**
Resting Pulse Rate:	
Nutrition:	
Journal:	

Date:	
Fitness:	**Stress Reduction:**
Resting Pulse Rate:	
Nutrition:	

Journal:

Date:	
Fitness:	**Stress Reduction:**
Resting Pulse Rate:	
Nutrition:	
Journal:	

Date:	
Fitness:	**Stress Reduction:**
Resting Pulse Rate:	
Nutrition:	
Journal:	

Date:	
Fitness:	**Stress Reduction:**
Resting Pulse Rate:	
Nutrition:	
Journal:	

Date:	
Fitness:	**Stress Reduction:**
Resting Pulse Rate:	
Nutrition:	
Journal:	

Date:	
Fitness:	**Stress Reduction:**
Resting Pulse Rate:	
Nutrition:	
Journal:	

Date:	
Fitness:	**Stress Reduction:**
Resting Pulse Rate:	
Nutrition:	

Journal:

_____

_____

_____

_____

_____

_____

_____

_____

_____

_____

_____

_____

_____

_____

_____

_____

Date:	
Fitness:	**Stress Reduction:**
Resting Pulse Rate:	
Nutrition:	

Journal:

Date:	
Fitness:	**Stress Reduction:**
Resting Pulse Rate:	
Nutrition:	
Journal:	

Date:	
Fitness:	**Stress Reduction:**
Resting Pulse Rate:	
Nutrition:	
Journal:	

Date:	
Fitness:	**Stress Reduction:**
Resting Pulse Rate:	
Nutrition:	

Journal:

Date:	
Fitness:	**Stress Reduction:**
Resting Pulse Rate:	
Nutrition:	

Journal:

Further Recommendations

There is an overwhelming amount of information on weight loss and dieting, most of which should be *ignored without question*. However, over the years I have found several sources of good information that fit well with the Cornerstone Concept and can be great resources for further learning and growth. To aid your journey, you might want to check out some of the following recommendations.

Diets Don't Work: Stop Dieting Become Naturally Thin Live a Diet-Free Life, Bob Schwartz (Breakthru Publishing). This is the best "diet" book I've ever seen.

The Heart of Addiction: A New Approach to Understanding and Managing Alcoholism and Other Addictive Behaviors, Lance M. Dodes (Quill). This book predominantly focuses on alcoholism, but also explores other addictions with a provocative theory that they are actually responses to perceived helplessness. It fits well with the paradigm concept.

Jane Siberry (self-titled CD, 1981) contains a song called *This Girl I Know* that lyrically captures the denial of an overweight woman making plans to lose weight. Although the Canadian artist's other CDs are readily available, this debut recording can be difficult to find but is worth the effort. If unavailable in stores, it can be ordered from her website, www.sheeba.ca

She's Come Undone, Wally Lamb (Pocket Books). A gripping novel that follows the life a girl battling life and a weight problem. A former *Oprah's Book Club* selection.

The Relaxation Response, Herbert Benson (HarperTorch). An excellent guide to meditation techniques.

The Seven Habits of Highly Effective People, Stephen Covey (Simon & Schuster). This famous book gives some great insights into paradigms and maintaining life priorities.

The Runner's Yoga Book, Jean Couch (Rodmell Press). The title of this book is somewhat misleading in that it is not just for runners. The format of this book makes it a great way to try yoga on your own. It is spiral bound so it can be opened easily on the floor, contains instructive photos, and classifies the stretches based on anatomy so that you can tailor make your own routine. It is a great way to try yoga if you are uncomfortable going to a class because of your weight.

Aerobics Program for Total Well-Being: Exercise, Diet, and Emotional Balance, Kenneth Cooper (Bantam). This is a classic book on the basic "aerobic effect" that creates dramatic changes in our metabolisms, sense of well-being, and overall physical fitness. It is a guide to virtually any type of fitness activity.

Galloway's Book on Running, Jeff Galloway (Shelter Publications). This book is a wonderful reference for someone interested trying running as a fitness activity. Jeff Galloway is a former Olympic athlete who has developed a common sense approach that has inspired thousands of runners. Jeff's marathon program is the one that I followed when I trained for my marathons. Also, visit his website (www.jeffgalloway.com) for lots of other useful ideas.

Authentic Happiness : Using the New Positive Psychology to Realize Your Potential for Lasting Fulfillment, Martin Seligman (Free Press). A unique approach to understanding and modifying your personal paradigm. There is an excellent supporting website (www.authentichappiness.org)

The Longevity Code, Zorba Paster (Three Rivers Press). This book makes a wonderful companion to the Cornerstone Concept. Public Radio host Dr. Zorba Paster's prescription for the Five Spheres of Wellness correlate nicely with the Four Cornerstones.

www.LosingIt.com, check the *LosingIt?* website for new information and updates, and to exchange ideas with others following the Cornerstone Concept!

About the Author

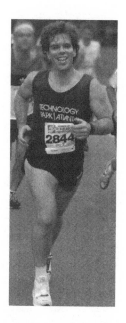

John Whitney was inspired to lose over 100 pounds of fat after attending Dr. Burt Bradley's class *The Psychology of Losing Weight and Never Finding It Again* in 1983. He has maintained the weight loss ever since without dieting, and continues to follow the Cornerstone Concept today. He has assisted Dr. Bradley with weight loss seminars, and wrote *Losing It?* to help others benefit from this unique approach to weight loss. He currently lives and teaches at a technical college in Wisconsin.

0-595-31573-9

Made in the USA
San Bernardino, CA
16 September 2015